Creative Yoga for Children

Creative Yoga for Children

Inspiring the Whole Child through Yoga, Songs, Literature, and Games

Forty Fun, Ready-to-Teach Lessons for Ages Four through Twelve

6 6 6 6 6

Adrienne Rawlinson

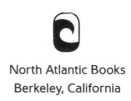

North Atlantic Books
Berkeley, California

Published by
North Atlantic Books
P.O. Box 12327
Berkeley, California 94712

Cover and book design by Brad Greene
Printed in the United States of America

Creative Yoga for Children: Inspiring the Whole Child through Yoga, Songs, Literature, and Games is sponsored by the Society for the Study of Native Arts and Sciences, a nonprofit educational corporation whose goals are to develop an educational and cross-cultural perspective linking various scientific, social, and artistic fields; to nurture a holistic view of arts, sciences, humanities, and healing; and to publish and distribute literature on the relationship of mind, body, and nature.

MEDICAL DISCLAIMER: The following information is intended for general information purposes only. Individuals should always see their health care provider before administering any suggestions made in this book. Any application of the material set forth in the following pages is at the reader's discretion and is his or her sole responsibility.

North Atlantic Books' publications are available through most bookstores. For further information, visit our website at www.northatlanticbooks.com or call 800-733-3000.

Library of Congress Cataloging-in-Publication Data

Rawlinson, Adrienne.
    Creative yoga for children: inspiring the whole child through yoga, songs, literature, and games / Adrienne Rawlinson.
        p. cm.
    ISBN 978-1-58394-554-4
    1. Hatha yoga for children. I. Title.
    RJ133.7.R39 2012
    613.7'046083—dc23
                                                    2012013562

1 2 3 4 5 6 7 8 9 SHERIDAN 18 17 16 15 14 13
Printed on recycled paper

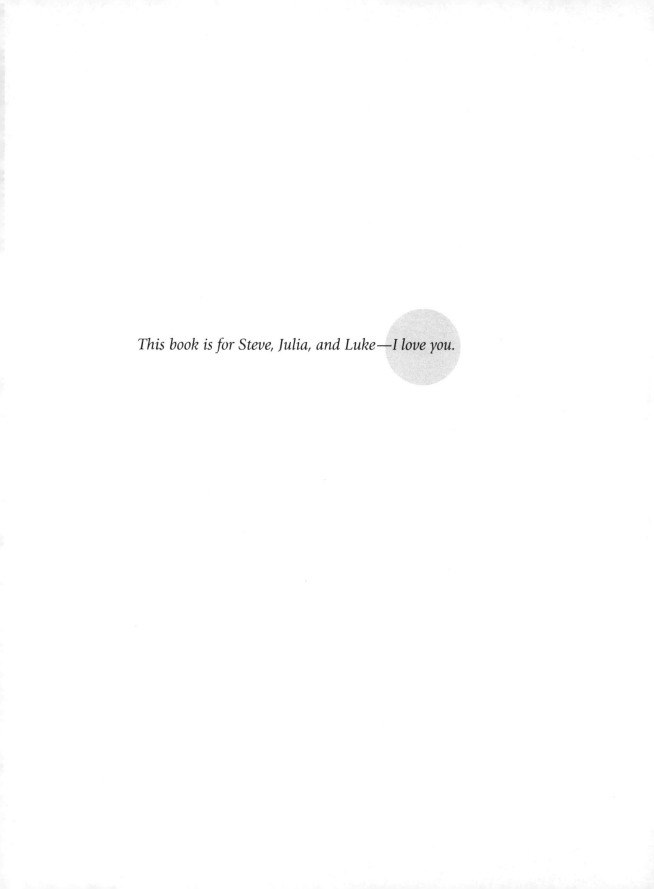

This book is for Steve, Julia, and Luke—I love you.

Acknowledgments

Thank you to Tom and Shirley Slee, Deb Cunningham, Karen Gardner, Jen Maclean, Alice Williams, Gary Senter, Melinda Clarke, Heather Lynn Berry, Jane French, Mayling Chung-Robinson, Gord Phippen, and a special thanks to my teacher, Maureen Rae. I would also like to thank the children in the book: Peri, Jordan, Logan, Erica, Cameron, Luke, Neeraj, and Julia.

Contents

Part I: Class Themes . . . 1

Four- to Six-Year-Olds

Part II: Class Themes . . . 91

Seven- to Nine-Year-Olds

Part III: Class Themes . . . 135

Ten- to Twelve-Year-Olds

Appendixes . . . 181

Introduction

Welcome to our program! *Creative Yoga for Children* is the product of many years of observing children in both yoga and Montessori classes. After teaching both Montessori and yoga, I have observed that the likenesses between the two are abundant. We know that yoga is the process of uniting the body and mind to become clearer and more centered. Montessori education is a holistic, hands-on approach to education that includes physical movement. So when combined, these two philosophies can only complement one another. This book merges the two practices into a fluid and beneficial program.

I have created a program that is completely accessible to all educators and parents, not just Montessori or yoga teachers. The classes are individually and logically laid out. They are divided into easy-to-use, age-appropriate parts (ages four to six, seven to nine, and ten to twelve). The classes help develop each child's conceptions of many subjects while remaining active and fun.

Like any learning environment, an engaging yoga class has a centering effect on children. It aids in constructing their confidence from the inside out. There is no huge emphasis on producing an end product, just a joy in the process. Children always feel successful in yoga; there is no competition, just an individual progression. Any child can enjoy yoga.

I believe in creating an environment that feeds a young child's need for order, movement, sensorial exploration, and language. This notion has been at the center of my yoga program. My teaching experiences have taught me that children's minds are at their optimal period for learning and absorbing the world's lessons and experiences before the age of twelve. These too are the key years for introducing them to the world of yoga.

Creative Yoga for Children provides a contemporary extension to traditional classroom activities. The child's understanding of specific educational topics is reinforced through a series of yoga poses, activities, and games. I know you will find this compilation of classes, developed from my years as a teacher and yoga instructor, to be beneficial to the children in your lives.

Move, Connect, and Learn

I remember my first taste of yoga. It was in our family room in Montreal in the 1970s. My mother would watch a morning yoga show, and I would rush to join her for our half hour together. The lady on the show doing poses fascinated me. I would giggle as I did the lotus, the crow, and other postures that introduced me to a whole new world. There were breathing exercises and even Sanskrit names for postures—how different! Of course, I was oblivious at the age of six to the monumental benefits of yoga. I just loved the time with my mom and the process of connecting and doing something together that put no pressure on either of us. This memory stands out vividly to me.

Now I realize that this little adventure mom and I shared left me with a feeling of acceptance, togetherness, and peace. Neither of us could actually do the poses, but this was irrelevant.

Years later I became a busy teacher and mother of my own two children. Yoga was no longer a part of my daily life. It was not until I felt a need to decompress and slow my busy life down that I took my first yoga class again in more than thirty years. The feeling of being right in the moment, of being soothed and satisfied, returned to me again. I wanted to pursue and explore my refound feelings.

I then immersed myself in my yoga practice. After obtaining my yoga teaching certification, I realized that I could apply yoga principles to the classroom. Kids had always been my comfort zone. The concept of harmonizing yoga with holistic education was the perfect fit!

I began to take various training workshops on teaching yoga to kids, all full of wonderful, usable ideas. After those workshops, it was time to get out there, culminate my training and experience, and give my children's yoga class a go.

I taught in churches, community centers, yoga studios, and even my own children's school as an extracurricular activity.

My enthusiasm grew, as did that of my students. My experience has always been that the key to success of any educational program is to methodically observe the needs of each individual child. So I learned from the kids by listening to and watching them. Consequently, I began to perfect my ideas and modify things I had planned to do, all in response to their input. Children, as we know, are infinitely wise, are honest, and have not yet constructed any walls to protect them from the world around them. I discovered that children were able to best learn concepts and ideas through movement and action. Through connection to movement and each other, children can learn complex concepts, such as our place in the universe, and have fun at the same time!

As I tried to find various programs and books to support my children's yoga practice, I realized that the existing resources available did not provide a "turnkey program," or a program I could immediately implement in the classroom. All the books I found required the reader to assemble classes from lists of poses and games. Subsequently, I developed classes for all age groups based on principles that can be implemented easily by anyone, saving them time in putting classes together.

While so many books I have used are helpful, I believe *Creative Yoga for Children* is uniquely user friendly. All my classes are laid out, step by step, from beginning to end. We have such limited time as educators and parents these days, so this book does all the planning for us.

My classes have evolved based on participant feedback. I have incorporated new poses suggested by the children, and our group discussions provided me with endless energy and ideas for new activities.

If any idea or activity in this collection can instill a feeling of connection and belonging within a few children, as my morning of television yoga sessions with my mom did in me, then my purpose is served.

If we all feel a part of one another, uniting us and instilling an appreciation of each other, then the connection is made. What more can we want for our children?

Creative Yoga for Children: From Preschool through Elementary

Where Do We Start?

We know that yoga is a wonderful tool used to promote the physical, emotional, and social development of children. Many programs offer this to our kids. However, the content of the *Creative Yoga for Children* classes not only addresses these fundamental needs of children but also offers a substantial innovation to an already established entity.

We begin our program by teaching such yoga fundamentals as poses, breathing techniques, and centering activities. Gradually, we blend these activities with those that also promote educational objectives. This is a very easy process, as the yogic and educational topics complement each other naturally.

The *Creative Yoga for Children* program is broken into three age groups: ages four to six, seven to nine, and ten to twelve.

Classes for Ages Four to Six

Children at this stage of development crave a logical order and flow to the classes every time. This makes them feel secure and confident. We allow time for them to repeat activities and poses. This repetition seals concepts in their minds. The props we use at this level appeal to the children's senses and their need to learn through touch and manipulation.

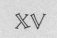

The collection of classes for our four- to six-year-olds promotes the following:

- Grace and courtesy
- Sensorial exploration and movement
- Coordination
- Balance
- Refinement of the writing hand
- Order
- Care of our environment, both indoors and outdoors
- Language
- Math
- Cooperation
- Artistic expression
- Self-care
- Physical health
- Self-awareness

Classes for Ages Seven to Nine

At this age children enter into a new plane of development. This is a more intellectual period than that of the four- to six-year-old child, and we now see a more reasoning, inquisitive personality emerge. The classes for this age group are designed to bring children into the world of abstract learning within a bigger social group that works together. These classes also offer more interactive group activities, supporting this need in each child.

Our classes for seven- to nine-year-olds classes build on these concepts and incorporate the following additional elements:

- Connection to those immediately around us
- Care of our planet
- Trust
- Karma yoga (giving back to the world and to each other)

- Empathy
- Intuition
- Language enrichment
- Gratitude
- Respect for the social group
- The ability to listen and to interpret ideas
- Imagination

Classes for Ages Ten to Twelve

The main goal of these classes is to develop a global vision within the child, who now wants to understand how the world functions and his or her place in it. Children in this age group are now able to analyze facts and generate new ideas and opinions. These classes leverage age-appropriate capabilities and will help children develop gratitude for the earth, the universe, and themselves.

Finally, our ten- to twelve-year-old children explore the following notions:

- Body changes
- Peer pressure
- Preparation for studying and the development of work habits
- Organization
- Community service
- Stress
- Reaching out beyond their inner circle of friends and family to the community

The Anatomy of a Class

It is comforting to a child to establish an ordered routine to the classes, just as order is so important in a child's home life.

Children take great satisfaction in knowing how each class is going to play out. This notion is a little less important as the child gets older, and of course we often have to improvise depending on the day, the children's moods, the weather, and just about any other variable!

All the classes will contain the following activities: Educational Elements, Props, Intention, Warm-up, Connect, Activity, Meditation, and Gratitude. Additionally, they may contain some other activities. The following is the complete list of activities that may be found in each class:

1. **Intention.** We discuss how we are feeling and then what we will focus on that day in class. For example, we might focus on the development of respect for nature, which we would explore by taking a trip to the park. Our goal might be to feel ultimately grateful for the natural world. We will revisit our intention whenever needed throughout the class.

2. **Warm-up.** This is a fun time of stretching and a series of interconnected poses or "vinyasas."

3. **Connect.** These are activities that stress how we all need one another—perhaps we might rub our hands together to create hot energy and connect our hands together in a circle, noticing how this feels. It is during this activity that we stress our need for human connection and how if we support and help one another, we can accomplish anything.

4. **Activity.** These are thematic activities based on the intention for the day's class and can involve large group games with music or dancing.

5. **Breath.** We introduce a new type of breathing technique or practice a cooling or heating breath.

6. **Arts and crafts.** This relates to our previous activities. For example, we may draw mandalas if we are discussing how to relax and focus, or we may make a clay model of the body if we are discussing muscles and bones.

7. **Book.** A book or story may be used to reinforce the intention of the class.

8. **Partner pose.** Partner poses are fun at any age, and we often introduce a new one in each class.

9. **Meditation.** This is often what kids look forward to and what they need the most. We relax, lie down on our mats, close our eyes, and enjoy a guided meditation for at least five minutes, accompanied by music. Some children enjoy a little foot and toe massage during this time, and I like to apply different scented lotions to add to the experience. They love this!

10. **Gratitude.** Once we come out of meditation, we take a few minutes to silently be grateful for something in our lives—perhaps our friends or our health. We sit for a moment and then end the class by repeating the word "Namaste," with our hands to our hearts. This means that we salute and honor each other.

In addition to these activities, each class will also contain reference to recommended "Props" and "Educational Elements." The "Props" are the recommended materials for each of the classes. These are items that I have found easy to obtain and may already be in your classroom. The educational elements are concepts that will be reinforced in each individual class.

Supporting all of these activities is music. This seems to be a key ingredient in all the classes, and I find that this is an ever-changing component. It is important to keep this element of the class alive and exciting. I recommend having different genres of music on hand. Children love to hear songs that they are familiar with and can dance to, as well as music for relaxation.

Part I:
Class Themes

Four- to Six-Year-Olds

1. Introduction to Yoga #1
2. Introduction to Yoga #2
3. Colors
4. The Sea
5. Winter
6. The Circus
7. Halloween
8. The Universe and Beyond
9. Going to the Park
10. Our Earth
11. The Holiday Season
12. Amazing Flowers
13. Mysteries
14. The Skeleton
15. Sounds and Words
16. Shapes and Numbers
17. Forest Life
18. Sniff, Touch, and Listen
19. Metamorphosis
20. Point of Arrival Class

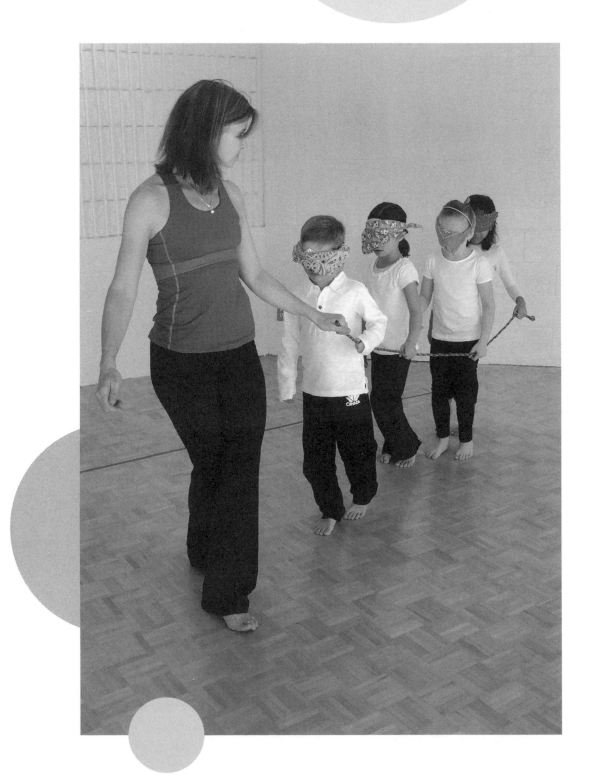

1.

Introduction to Yoga #1

Four- to Six-Year-Olds

Educational Elements: language development (prana, vinyasa, namaste), freedom of movement throughout, order (the format and routine that each class will follow), sensorial exploration (the concept of the poses, introduced concretely through the animal objects)

Props: Hoberman sphere or a sea sponge, animal bag, yoga mats, chimes, music, book (*Brown Bear, Brown Bear, What Do You See?* by Bill Martin Jr. and Eric Carle), small stuffed animals, body lotion

Intention: Begin by laying out your mats in whatever formation your space allows for (a circle works nicely). Welcome the children and ask them to sit on their mats. Explain that their mat is their special place where they will practice yoga, and if they don't feel comfortable doing the exercises, then they can observe from their mats. Today the intention will be to learn about yoga. Have a discussion about this. Ask the kids what they think yoga is. Explain how it is an ancient philosophy developed in India. Yogis developed poses or "asanas" to help their bodies feel good and their minds be clear. We can use yoga at work, at school, and in other parts of our lives whenever we need to relax and take a moment for ourselves. Introduce the chimes and explain that they will be used to signal the end of an activity, at which point the children are to quietly return to their mats and listen. Have the children close their eyes, ring the chimes, and when they can't hear or feel any vibration anymore, they can raise their hands. Experiment with this little activity.

Time: Five to Ten Minutes

Warm-Up: Pick two or three new poses from the pose object bag and demonstrate them. Have the children try them. Incorporate them into a little flow to music, naming each pose as you go. The children will mirror you. Make it fun without emphasizing that they should do the poses correctly; tell them to just give them a try, remembering to breathe in and out while doing them.

Time: Five to Ten Minutes

Connect: Group balance. Explain how we will connect in all our classes. Emphasize that we are all important to our group and that we help and need each other. Have the children practice a connection activity. Ask them to take hold of their classmates' wrists on either side of them in the circle. Tell them to all stand up together. Following that, tell them to balance on one foot, and then have them switch to the other foot. They should stay holding on to each other as they all sit back down. Bring to their attention how you helped each other do this. Now ask the children to rub their hands together very quickly to

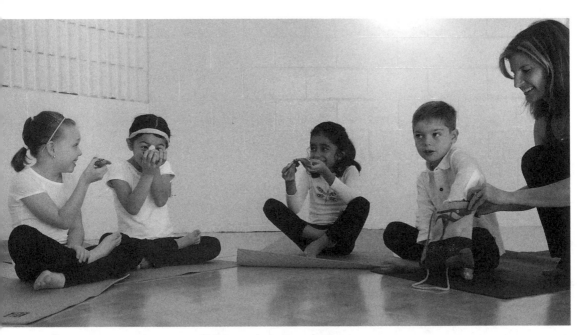

Figure 1.1. Children choosing a pose

create friction, and after a minute, have them place each palm almost up against the palm of the child on either side of them. Ask them if they can feel this energy between their hands and explain how it connects us all.

Time: Five to Ten Minutes

Activity: Introduction to poses. Bring out the pose object bag. Pass it around and, with their eyes closed, have each child reach in and choose one—no peeking! Demonstrate and name the pose each child chooses and invite everyone to join in on the pose. Help those who need it, but precision is not the key here. The children can do their own version of the pose. Older children will happily help the younger ones. When everyone has chosen, lay all the poses out so the class can see them. Tell the kids, "We will now do a little flow of all the poses put together." Use music and go slowly. Demonstrate the flow and name each pose as you go; the children will follow you through it. Afterward tell them that they have just demonstrated a "vinyasa." Let them try the poses on their own for a few minutes before ringing the chimes.

Time: Approx. Fifteen Minutes

Breath: The breathing ball. Take out your small expandable or "Hoberman" sphere (or a small sea sponge) and explain that it is your breathing ball. Demonstrate that when we breathe, our bellies and lungs expand, as the ball does, and as we exhale, they get smaller, also like the ball. Pass the sphere to the children and have them pass it around; each student can have a turn expanding it as he or she inhales and contracting as he or she exhales. Explain that "prana" in yoga is our life force, and it moves through us and sustains us. We must try to breathe well and deeply all the time.

Time: Five to Ten Minutes

Book: As you read this to the children, tell them they can demonstrate the poses in the book as they hear them—most of these poses they have seen today. Use *Brown Bear, Brown Bear, What Do You See?* by Bill Martin Jr. and Eric Carle.

Time: Five to Ten Minutes

Meditation: Ring the chimes. Explain that they will come back to their mats and relax. The children can lie back on their mats. Tell them to sink into their mats as if they are butter melting on toast. Tell them their mat is now their magic carpet. Lay a little stuffed toy animal on each child's belly. This is their passenger that will rise up and down on their belly as they breathe in and out. Tell them to be still so their passenger won't fall off. Continue on with a story of flying over the world on a magic carpet, looking down and noticing mountains, cities, oceans, and other things. Engage their imaginations. Give the

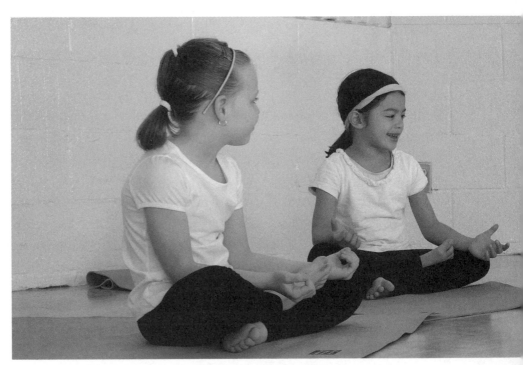

Figure 1.2. Exploring the breath with the breathing ball

children who agree to it a little toe rub with mildly scented lotion while you are speaking. They will love this.

Time: Seven to Ten Minutes

Gratitude: Ring the chimes softly, and tell the children to gradually stretch and roll over onto one side. Ask them to come up to a seated position with their hands to their hearts. Tell them that this hand position is called a "mudra." Ask them to close their eyes and take a moment to silently be thankful for everything and everyone around them and for anyone else they love in their lives (things to be grateful for are many, so each class will differ in this way). Then repeat the word "namaste" to them and explain that it means that the "light inside of me bows down to the light inside of you." Have them repeat it. End of class.

Time: Five to Ten Minutes

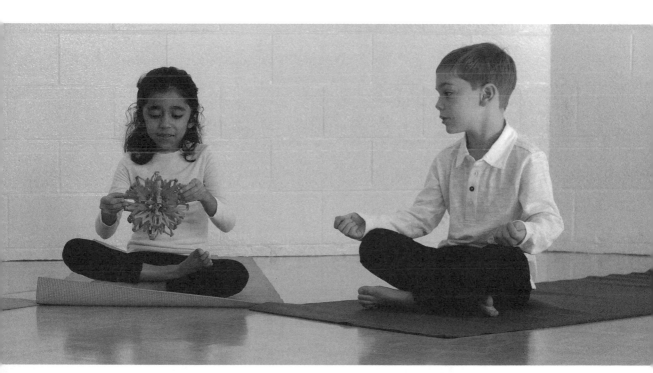

2.

Introduction to Yoga #2

Four- to Six-Year-Olds

Educational Elements: Sensorial exploration, freedom of movement, familiarity with the order of the class, freedom of choice to participate at the child's own pace and capacity, language development, coordination and refinement of movement, grace and courtesy within the group

Props: Herbal eye pillows (one for each child), selection of pose objects, hula hoops, yoga mats, book (*Hairy Maclary's Rumpus at the Vet* by Lynley Dodd), chimes, selection of music, foot lotion

Intention: Having prepared the environment for them, invite the children to choose a mat in the circle to sit on. They can move freely until everyone is ready. Greet the children by ringing the chimes. Welcome them to yoga and ask them to listen and sit comfortably. Tell them that for this class, you all will have another look at the poses from the first class. During these first few classes, the emphasis is on having the children get comfortable with the routine of the program and to familiarize them with the poses. Answer their questions as they arise. Remind them that you will ring the chimes between activities.

Time: Five to Ten Minutes

Warm-Up: Tell the children that you are going to make a pizza together. Have them sit up on their mats with legs stretched out in a V shape to represent a slice of pizza. Ask the children what they need to do first to make the slice of pizza—perhaps some dough. Demonstrate rolling out the dough, throwing it up in the air, and stretching it out. Ask the children for ingredients—they will have lots of ideas. As they call out things like pepperoni, cheese, and mushrooms, demonstrate how the toppings are chopped, diced, stretched out, and placed all over the pizza. Their bodies will stretch, move, and warm right up. Make this fun and active. When the pizza is finished, have them pretend to eat it.

Time: Approx. Ten Minutes

Connect: Energy rub. Ask the children to inch toward the front of their mats, and tell them that they are going to connect to each other and pass their energy from one person to the next. Have them rub their hands together first, very quickly to create friction, and then have them all join hands. Emphasize that the energy they are passing will be shared among them for everyone's benefit. Start by squeezing the child's hand beside you and have them then squeeze the child's hand beside them, and so on until the squeeze has returned around the circle back to you. Do this a few times, having different children start the "squeeze."

Time: Approx. Five Minutes

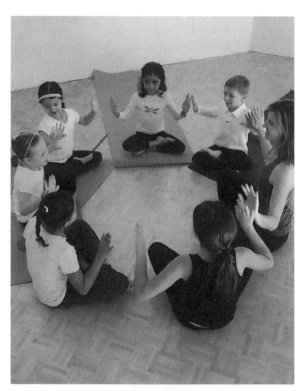

Figure 1.3. Connecting with energy

Activity: Hula hoop dancing. Have as many large hula hoops scattered around your room as there are children. Bring out the pose bag from last class and include in it the poses from last time as well as a few new ones. Add new poses in each time until the children are familiar with all of them. Pass the bag around and have the children each choose an object (pose) from the bag. Name them and demonstrate them as you go. The children can then place their pose object into any hula hoop they choose and stand inside the hoop. Play music at different intervals. Explain that they can dance and move any way they like when they hear the music, and when the music stops, they can find a hoop and practice doing the pose that is in it. Repeat these steps, having them choose a different hoop at the halt of the music each time. See how the children are managing with this. If the children need assistance with the poses, the older ones can partner up with the younger ones. Ring the chimes when the children have had enough.

Time: Ten to Fifteen Minutes

Breath: Straw breathing. When the children return to their mats, it is a good time for a cooling breath exercise. Tell then to relax and stick out their tongues, forming a straw shape with them. They can pretend to sip lemonade or their favorite drink with the straw, close their mouths, and exhale slowly out their noses. Have them repeat this several times. They can even pretend to squeeze lemons with their feet to make lemonade, squeezing them into their

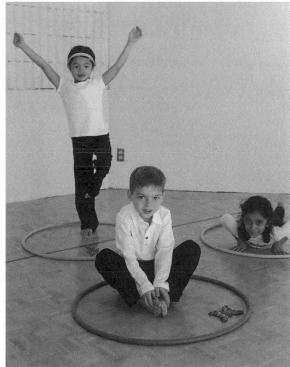

Figure 1.4. Hula hoop dancing

imaginary glass that they drink from. Ask them if they feel cool after this exercise.

Time: Approx. Five Minutes

Book: *Hairy Maclary's Rumpus at the Vet* by Lynley Dodd. This is a hilarious story of a dog's visit to the vet and the animals that he meets there. The children can demonstrate the animal poses they have done in the class as they hear them in the book.

Time: Approx. Ten Minutes

Meditation: The children can now settle down on their mats for savasana, or meditation. Have them place their arms down by their sides with their palms open to the sky, eyes closed. Lay an herbal eye pillow over each child's eyes very gently. Some will not be interested in using this and some will love it. Dim the lights and put on soft music. You can tell the children that they are tall, strong mountains that have been around for millions of years. They have seen many things come and go. The wind has blown over them, trees have grown on them, storms have come and gone, and different animals have climbed up and lived on them. Through it all they have been steady and strong, still and quiet. Add your own elements to the story.

Time: Five to Ten Minutes

Gratitude: Ring the chimes softly and tell the children, in their own time, to gradually stretch and roll over onto one side. Have them move to a seated position with their hands to their hearts. Ask them to silently give thanks for your time together and for being healthy, happy, and loved. Ask them to take a moment whenever they can to silently feel grateful. Repeat the phrase "Namaste, the light within me bows down to the light inside of you."

Time: Five to Ten Minutes

3.

Colors

Four- to Six-Year-Olds

Educational Elements: Visual discrimination of color, freedom of choice and freedom of movement, cooperation, and repetition of poses they have learned to solidify the concepts

Props: Supply of multicolored feathers; several dryer sheets; red, yellow, and blue food coloring; newspaper to spread underneath; several pipe cleaners cut in half; chimes; music; pose object bag

Intention: Have the children settle on their mats, ring the chimes, and welcome them to yoga. The intention for this class will be to notice and be mindful of the colors around us. They can discuss their favorite colors. They can discuss colors they associate with their moods or the seasons. Try to engage them in a little discussion and make them feel comfortable.

Time: Approx. Five Minutes

Warm-Up: Pick two or three new poses from the pose object bag and demonstrate them. Have the children try them. Incorporate them into a little flow to music, naming each pose as you go. The children will mirror you. Make it fun without emphasizing that they should do the poses correctly; tell them to just give them a try, remembering to breathe in and out while doing them.

Time: Approx. Ten Minutes

Connect: Web of compliments. Take out a ball of multicolored wool. Hold onto it and say something wonderful about one child in the circle, for example, "John is a smart guy." Hold the end of the wool with one hand and toss the ball of wool to John. He will catch it, pay a compliment to another child in the circle, hold his end of the wool, and toss the ball to that child. This continues on until everyone has had a turn and the ball of wool can come back to you. Invite the children to hold on tight to their wool and slowly stand up with it. This creates a beautiful "rainbow-colored web of compliments" for them to admire. They can raise it up and down a few times and release it.

Time: Approx. Ten Minutes

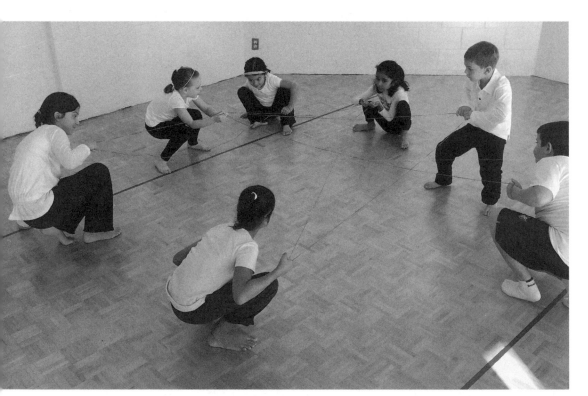

Figure 1.5. Web of compliments

Activity: Color dancing. Choose some lively dance music to put on. Scatter the objects from the pose bag on the floor. All the objects will have a separate color of their own (e.g., the blue dolphin, the red plough, the green snake). Have the children dance to the music and then stop as you turn the music off. Ask the children to pick up the object nearest to them. Call out a color, for example, red, and whichever child has the red object will do that pose. The others may do the red-object pose it as well. When the children place their objects down again, the music comes back on. You might want to ask them to jump to the music instead of dancing, or jog to it, or walk on their tiptoes—just play it by ear. When you stop the music, call out a different color. Continue this until everyone has a turn and most of the colors are called.

Time: Ten to Fifteen Minutes

Breath: Bird breath. Scatter some different colored feathers around in your circle. Tell the children that the class will be doing bird poses today. Assign colors to different birds. For example, the flamingo feathers are pink, the crow feathers are black, the pigeon feathers are grey, and the eagle feathers are brown. Have the children pick up two feathers they want. If they have a pink and a brown, for example, ask them to do the flamingo and the eagle pose. After they have experimented with this, invite them to put their feathers back on the ground and to kneel down in front of them. Ask them to use their biggest breath, in through the nose and out through the mouth, to blow the feathers all into the middle of the circle. When they have done this, they will have made a rainbow of feathers. Ask them what type of bird would have all these different colors. They will have lots of ideas.

Time: Approx. Ten Minutes

Arts and Crafts: Making butterflies. Pass out two fabric sheets to each child. Demonstrate with your own sheets how when blue and yellow are mixed, they create green. Using food coloring, drop blue and green drops onto the sheets to make the new color. Drop a few red drops with yellow to create orange. Then mix a few red drops with blue to create purple. Let the children try this now. When they are finished, help them twist a little pipe cleaner around the middle of their sheets to make the body in the center of the butterfly. Make sure to put newspaper down underneath their artwork!

Time: Ten to Fifteen Minutes

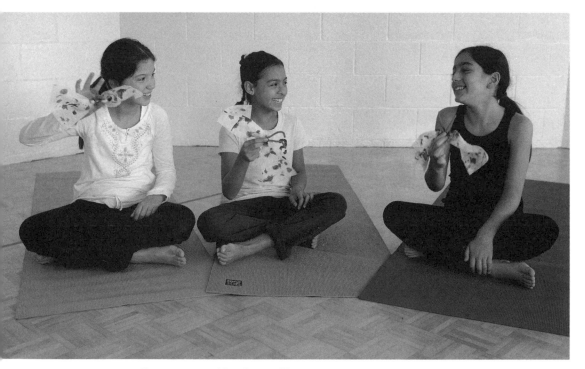

Figure 1.6. Making butterflies

Meditation: The children can lie down on their mats after you have put the artwork to the side. Dim the lights and put on soft music. You can offer them herbal eye pillows if they would like them. Begin a little story about going on a trip over the rainbow. Tell the children to imagine that they are riding on their mats up into the sky, feeling light as a feather. They will stop at each color. As they arrive at the color red, ask them to imagine a red apple, a red rose, a red heart, and so on. Ask them to continue gliding on to the next color and imagine what they see. At the end of the whole rainbow, tell them that they are gliding back down to Earth and softly landing.

Time: Approx. Seven to Ten Minutes

Gratitude: Ask the children to slowly stretch and bring their knees into their chest, wrap their arms around their legs, and rock from side to side. Tell them that they are giving themselves a hug. Gradually, have them return to the sitting position with their hands to their hearts. Ask them to close their eyes and silently be grateful for all the beauty that surrounds us in our lives and colors our world. Ask them to remember to always stop and appreciate what they see. End with "Namaste, the light in me bows down to the light in you."

Time: Five to Ten Minutes

4.

The Sea

Four- to Six-Year-Olds

Educational Elements: Language enrichment, sensorial exploration of all materials, artistic expression, grace and courtesy within the group, freedom of movement

Props: pose object bag that includes an octopus, a dolphin, a fish, a jellyfish, a seal, a crab, a starfish, a mermaid, a boat, and an alligator; construction paper; stamps; stamp pads; sand; book (*The Rainbow Fish* by Marcus Pfister); chimes; music; hula hoops; foot lotion; herbal eye pillows

Intention: Gather the children and tell them that the class is going on a sea excursion. You might begin by saying, "Did you know that two-thirds of the world is covered in water? Has anyone here been to the ocean before?" Have a little discussion about the children's experiences with the ocean.

Time: Five to Ten Minutes

Warm-Up: Ask the children to begin with a little flow, or "vinyasa." Tell them, "Let's pretend that we are inside a shell. Let's make ourselves small, now let's grow bigger, bigger, and burst out! Raise your arms up to the sky, breathe in as you raise one arm to the sky, and breathe out as you bring your arm down. Now let's reach the other arm to the sky as we breathe in." Repeat this breath sequence a few more times. Then proceed with a flow sequence that the children can follow. Include poses they have all seen before.

Time: Five to Ten Minutes

19

Creative Yoga for Children

Connect: Human swirl. Tell the children that you are going to make a "human swirl," like a whirlpool in the ocean. Talk about whirlpools a little. Ask everyone to join hands and then let go of one child's hand as you twirl. Turn around and around and draw the children around with you, as if you are winding them around a spool of thread. Go slowly, and when you are all wound up together, ask the last child on the outside to begin to "undo" the swirl, unraveling everyone. Try this again, having other children start the swirl off.

Time: Five to Ten Minutes

Activity 1: Tunnel swim. Have the children hold a hula hoop each out in front of them, creating a sort of "tube" or "tunnel." Have a bag of sea creature poses available and ask the first child to choose one. The child may choose, for example, a crab and can then move through the tunnel of hoops as a crab would. The first child rejoins the line of children and takes the next child's hula hoop. The next child then

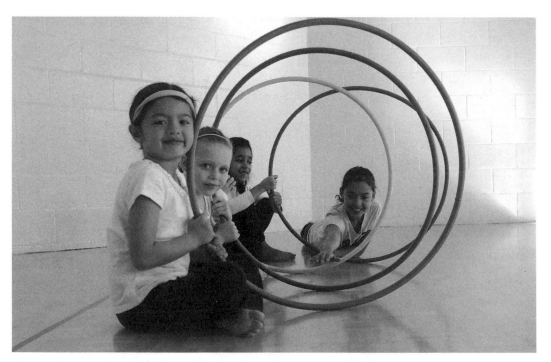

Figure 1.7. Tunnel swim

takes a turn choosing a sea creature and moving through the tunnel. Repeat this cycle until every child has had several turns.

Time: Approx. Fifteen Minutes

Activity 2: A sea voyage. Ask the children to spread out and find their own space. Begin telling them a little story and ask them to act out the story with poses and gestures. Ask them to board their boats, row out to see, and dive off, going underwater as scuba divers do. Tell them to take big breaths through their air tanks. Journey around, observing sharks, jellyfish, crabs, octopi, and other sea creatures. Observe whales and dolphins near the surface. Add in your own elements to the story. Finally, have the children board their boats again and row to shore. Finish by ringing your chimes and have them return to their mats.

Time: Approx. Fifteen Minutes

Arts and Crafts: Seascapes. Tell the children that they now going to make what they saw when they were on their underwater adventure. Using stamps of various sea creatures and different-colored stamp pads, have the children design their underwater world. They can simply draw the creatures if stamps are unavailable. They can also apply glue to the bottom of their construction paper and adhere a little sand to it, creating a very sensorial surface for the bottom of their "ocean."

Time: Approx. Fifteen Minutes

Book: *The Rainbow Fish* by Marcus Pfister is a nice way to finish off the class. The children can enjoy doing the poses of the characters in the book as they listen to the story.

Time: Five Minutes

Partner Pose: Octopus. Choose a child to demonstrate the "octopus" partner pose with (see "Partner Pose Guide" in appendix). Have the children pair off and try the pose themselves.

Time: Approx. Five Minutes

Meditation: Bring the children to their mats for final meditation/relaxation. Offer them eye pillows if they would like. Have them lie down, eyes closed, in whatever position feels nice for them.

Some children will curl up on their sides while others will lie in a traditional savasana pose on their backs. Dim the lights and turn on soft music. Tell the children to imagine that their mat is a submarine and they are lying safe in it. The submarine then submerges and floats down toward the bottom of the sea, lower and lower. Perhaps they see colorful fish swimming by, or a blue dolphin waving at them, or sea turtles swimming. Add your own elements to this story. Finally, have the submarine resurface. Apply foot lotion to children who may want this.

Time: Five to Ten Minutes

Gratitude: Have the children slowly stretch and roll over to one side. When they finally sit up, try a new mudra (hand position), the "OK" mudra (refer to OK mudra, page 201) with both hands resting on each knee. Ring the chimes softly and ask them to close their eyes and take a moment to be grateful for the things in their lives that they love and for the other children all around them. Then repeat together, "Namaste, the light in me bows down to the light within you."

Time: Five to Ten Minutes

5.
Winter

Four- to Six-Year-Olds

Educational Elements: Sensorial exploration of zoology, freedom of movement, language development, a familiar sequence of activities catering to the child's need for order

Props: Cotton balls, construction paper, colored pencils, yoga mats, foot lotion (optional), Tibetan singing bows, music, hibernation book (*The Animals' Winter Sleep* by Lynda Graham-Barber and Nancy Carol Willis)

Intention: Welcome the children and have them sit on their mats. Introduce them to listening to a singing bowl. A singing bowl is a bronze bowl used in yoga to assist in meditation and to signify the commencement of an activity. They can listen to a singing bowl's sound when an activity is ending and it is time for more instructions. Ring the bowl for them and have them close their eyes and listen—they will want to have a turn trying to ring this! Now explain that they are going to have fun in the snow today and talk about things they associate with winter. Perhaps talk about what happens to animals and plants in the winter.

Time: Five to Ten Minutes

Warm-Up: Tell the children that it is a very cold day and that they can pretend to be asleep under their warm covers on their mats. After a few minutes, they can pull off their blankets, step out of bed, and open the curtains. The sun shines in, so they can do a few sun salutations, and then a little flow of poses.

Time: Approx. Five Minutes

Connect: Making snowballs. Sitting back on their mats, the children can rub their hands together vigorously for a minute and then gradually pull them apart, feeling the "energy" they have created. Ask them to shape that energy into a snowball, lifting it up and down. Finally, have them throw it away, creating a "warmth" that connects everyone and preparing them to go out in the snow.

Time: Approx. Five Minutes

Activity: A winter day. Tell the children to imagine that now you are all going to get dressed to go out. Go through the body parts with them, asking what they need first to put on their heads, their ears, around their necks, and so on. They will act out getting dressed and give you all their ideas. When you are finished, tell them you are going out—put on music and have the children venture out into the imaginative snowy world. Have them feel the wind as they travel through the snow. Suggest that they make snow angels. Suggest that they roll themselves into snowballs. Suggest that they become snow ploughs, in plough pose, and plough the roads. The kids will give you more suggestions. Continue along in this way on your snow adventure. Then ring the singing bowl and invite them to come back to their mats, shake off the snow, and mimic taking off their winter clothes.

Time: Approx. Ten Minutes

Breath: Snow shoveling. Hand out cotton balls, making sure each child gets several. Suggest that the class build a snow fort in the center of the circle, but the children will have to use breath energy to move the snow in front of them. Tell them to feel their bellies rise as they inhale and lower as they exhale, blowing the snow into the middle. Afterward, they can admire their fort.

Time: Approx. Five Minutes

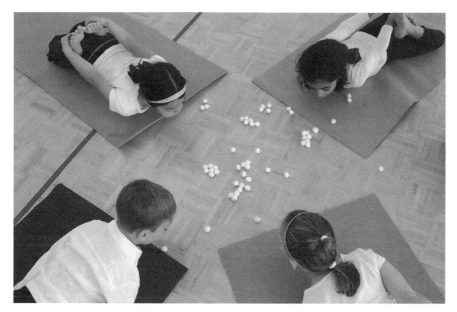

Figure 1.8. Snow shoveling

Arts and Crafts: Hibernating animals. Invite the children to draw pictures showing three different types of creatures hibernating. Provide each child a piece of paper divided into three sections for this craft. Discuss everyone's drawings afterward.

Time: Ten to Fifteen Minutes

Book: Invite them to relax as you read a book about animal hibernation, *The Animals' Winter Sleep* by Lynda Graham-Barber and Nancy Carol Willis. They can sit in their favorite pose.

Time: Five to Ten Minutes

Meditation: Ring the singing bowl and have the children come to their mats, relax, and lie down comfortably. Have them close their eyes as you turn on peaceful music. Tell them that now they are hibernating too. They can imagine being their favorite creature and that they are getting ready for a long rest. They are melting into their beds for the winter. Their breath should be soft and slow. Add your own elements to this story. After their "sleep," invite them to slowly wake up because spring has arrived. The children "wake up" by stretching on their backs, reaching as far is they can with their fingers and toes. Complete the meditation by rolling over and coming up to a seated position.

Time: Five to Ten Minutes

Gratitude: Have them try a new mudra today, perhaps bringing their ring finger to their thumb for the Earth mudra. Tell them that doing this mudra makes them feel strong (refer to Earth mudra, page 201).

Ask them to silently be grateful for their strong, healthy bodies today and for their ability to do this fun yoga practice together. Repeat, "Namaste, the light in me bows down to the light inside of you."

Time: Five to Ten Minutes

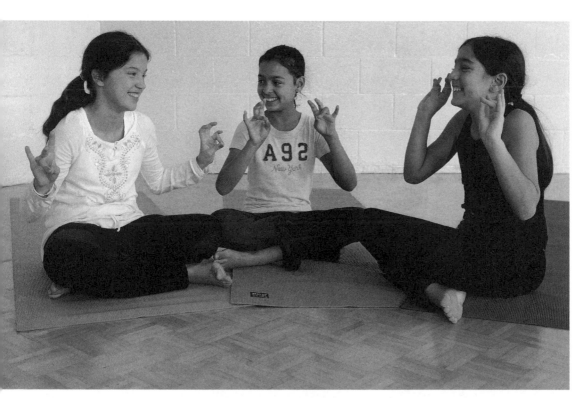

Figure 1.9. Gratitude: Earth mudra

6.

The Circus

Four- to Six-Year-Olds

Educational Elements: Freedom of movement, language development, familiar sequence of activities catering to child's need for order, artistic expression, development of the writing hand

Props: Construction paper with outlines of blank faces on it, colored pencils or markers, book (*When Sophie Gets Angry—Really, Really Angry . . .* by Molly Bang), pose object bag, foot lotion, yoga mats, stuffed animals

Intention: Gather the children on their mats, ring the chimes or the singing bowl, and welcome them to yoga. Tell them that today they will be going on a circus trip. Discuss this with the students, asking them what they think they will see. Ask them about their experiences at the circus.

Time: Five to Ten Minutes

Warm-Up: Introduce the seal, the elephant, and the lion pose from the pose object bag if the children aren't already familiar with it. Have them practice these three poses as you demonstrate them. Then have the children stand up and do a little warm-up flow of poses, starting with a sun salutation.

Time: Approx. Five Minutes

Connect: House of mirrors. Tell the children that as they arrive at the circus, they are entering through the fun house, which is full of funny-shaped mirrors. Pair the children off and invite them to try "mirroring" each other. They face their partners, with one child leading the movements. They can start with little hand movements, then facial expressions, then full walking movements—whatever they can think of. Then have them switch, allowing the second child to lead the sequence.

Time: Five to Ten Minutes

Activity: The circus show. Ask the children to scatter around the room and spread out. Then begin to tell them a story of the circus, having them act it out. You can have them watch the man on the flying trapeze, the lions, the clowns, the seals, the elephants, the tightrope walker, and the jugglers. Link your story to some of the poses the children have learned. Finally, have them leave the circus, come home to their mats, and relax in their favorite pose.

Time: Ten Minutes

Breath: Volcano breath. Explain to the children that when they feel impatient or upset, a great breath to make them feel better is the volcano breath. Have them squat down in the shape of a volcano. Tell them hot lava is rising up as they inhale, and as they stand up they can exhale, reaching up with their arms, making all the lava shoot out of the volcano. Repeat this a few times.

Time: Five Minutes

Arts and Crafts: Funny faces. Invite the children to make faces. Have several blank faces drawn on a piece of paper for each child, and ask them to draw expressions on the faces showing how they felt during their trip to the circus today. They might draw a tired face for their end of the day, a scared face for when they saw the tigers, a happy face when they saw the clowns, and so on. Discuss all their expressions and have them share their pictures.

Time: Ten Minutes

Book: Explain to the kids that a lot of emotions came up when they drew their faces. Read them a book called *When Sophie Gets Angry— Really, Really Angry . . .* by Molly Bang and talk about the emotions that it shows.

Time: Ten Minutes

Partner Pose: Shoulder wheels. Have the children group into pairs. Have each pair stand side to side about two feet apart holding each other's wrist. Each pair slowly rotates their shoulders forward, making a complete circle with their hands. Repeat this sequence several times in the forward and backward directions. Have the children change sides and repeat (partner pose 2, page 189).

Time: Five to Ten Minutes

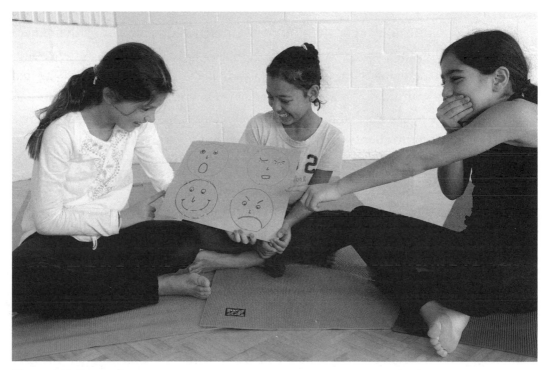

Figure 1.10. Funny faces

Meditation: Have the children return to their mats, relax, lie down, and close their eyes as they hear the chimes or singing bowl. Dim the lights and play tranquil music. Use lotion to rub their feet (optional) or lay little stuffed animals on their bellies, telling them that they are taking their animal friend on a ride down a lazy river. They must keep the animal safe by breathing very evenly and slowly and being still. Tell the children that they are lying on soft pillows on a boat that is gliding down a windy, blue river. There are beautiful trees and flowers along the river banks and green, shiny grass. Talk about things we see along the river bank, like rabbits, raccoons, deer, and so on. Talk about things in the river like fish, otters, and frogs. Add your own elements to the story, and finally, have the boat glide into the shore where they can step out.

Time: Five to Ten Minutes

Gratitude: Invite the children to stretch and maybe bring their knees into their chests and wrap their arms around themselves and their animal, giving themselves a hug. Gradually, they can come up to a seated position and try a new mudra called water mudra that will help balance the water that is in our bodies (see water mudra, page 201). Ask them to silently be grateful for their families and to think one by one of each member of their family and why they love them. Conclude with "Namaste, the light within me honors the light within you."

Time: Five to Ten Minutes

7.

Halloween

Four- to Six-Year-Olds

Educational Elements: Freedom of movement and choice, sensorial exploration, language development, artistic expression, sequence of activities that fulfills need for order

Props: Toy frog; lily pad made of construction paper; orange, black, and white modeling clay; book (*I Know an Old Lady Who Swallowed a Bat* by Lucille Colandro); appropriate music for Halloween; yoga mats; lotion; herbal eye pillows

Intention: Invite the children to sit on their mats. You might use a gong today instead of chimes, explaining to the children that when they hear the gong, it means the same as the chimes of the singing bowl. Have them try the gong out for themselves. Explain that this is a special Halloween adventure class. They will meet some scary and some funny creatures on their journey today. Discuss the children's experiences with Halloween, a holiday they often love even more than Christmas.

Time: Five to Ten Minutes

Warm-Up: Ask the children to sit cross-legged or to kneel on their mats. Tell them they are making a witch's brew for a Halloween party. Pretend you are holding a huge stick and stir an imaginary pot, stirring in one direction first and then reversing it. Ask the children for suggestions of what to put in the pot—perhaps frogs, spiders, newts, and so on. Afterward, do a little vinyasa, introducing a crescent moon pose from the pose object bag. This is the moon that will be out on Halloween night.

Time: Eight to Ten Minutes

Connect: Transport the frog. Use a toy frog and ask the children to work together to transport this frog to his lily pad. The children can spread out from one end of the room to the other. One child then balances the frog on his belly and proceeds to crab walk slowly over to another child, placing it on that child's belly. That child then does the same and so on. When the frog has gone to all the children, the last child can crab walk the frog over to the lily pad.

Time: Five to Ten Minutes

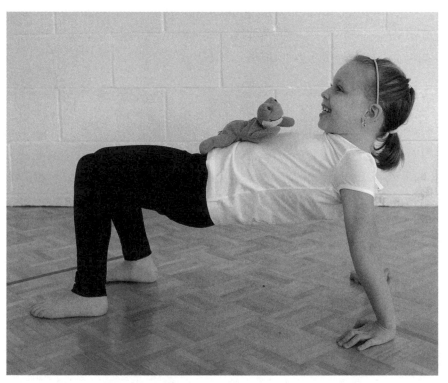

Figure 1.11. Transport the frog

Activity: A Halloween story. Tell the children a Halloween story that they can act out. Some children can play the part of the pumpkins, some can be cats, and the rest can be ghosts (dividing the group evenly into thirds). Have the children spread out in the room and practice how their character might look and move. Begin the story:

> Once upon a time there were a group of ghosts, pumpkins, and black cats. It was Halloween and they all woke up and stretched in the morning. They saluted the sun as it rose in the sky. Then they all set off for Halloween Town for a big party that night. The pumpkins left first because they were the slowest, rolling across the fields. Then the cats left, sprinting and pouncing all the way. Finally, the ghosts started on the path, flying gracefully across the sky. They all had to stop suddenly because they had reached a mountain that they had to climb. The ghosts had no problem and flew right up. The pumpkins, however, kept rolling down every time they tried to make the big climb. So the cats kindly pushed them up the mountain until they reached the top. The pumpkins then rolled quickly down the other side, chased by the cats. All the creatures reached a river that they all had to cross in their own way. The ghosts again flew over the water easily. The cats hated the water, so they hitched a ride on the pumpkins, which floated across the river like boats. Finally they all reached Halloween Town where they joined the party— they bobbed for apples, laughed, and danced. Above them they saw the huge crescent moon in the dark sky.

The children will add their own elements to this story.

Time: Approx. Ten to Fifteen Minutes

Breath: Back breathing. Ask the children to come into child's pose and imagine that they are big swamp toads. Participants can get into child's pose by kneeling with their head in their laps and their hands extend over their knees. As they inhale, tell them to feel the sides of their backs expand outward, like the side of a frog's neck does. You can ask them to do this with a partner, having one person be the breathing toad and the other feeling their partner's back expand as they breathe, using the palms of their hands.

Time: Five to Ten Minutes

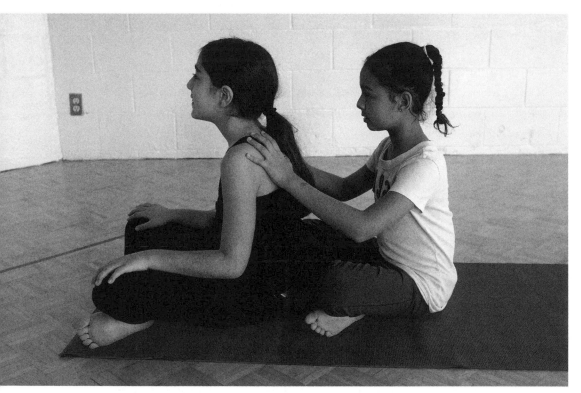

Figure 1.12. Back breathing

Arts and Crafts: Sculptures. Invite the children to make modeling clay versions of the pumpkins, cats, or ghosts that were in the story. They can make other Halloween creatures if they choose to.

Time: Ten to Fifteen Minutes

Book: *I Know an Old Lady Who Swallowed a Bat* by Lucille Colandro. The children can act out the creatures in the book.

Time: Ten Minutes

Meditation: Have the children relax on their mats now, using your gong to initiate the end of the activity. As they close their eyes, offer them an herbal eye pillow if they like. Foot lotion is also optional. Begin to tell them a story of a witch's flight over the world on Halloween night. Have them pretend that they are flying beside her on their flying mats. Point out what the witch sees below, perhaps houses dressed up in Halloween decorations, children trick-or-treating, or a pumpkin patch, adding in your own elements to the story. Finally, have the witch return to her home, coming in for a landing and going to sleep after a long Halloween night.

Time: Eight to Ten Minutes

Gratitude: Have the children stretch, roll over slowly, and come up to a seated position. A nice mudra for them to try is their middle finger touching their thumb (refer to tall house mudra, pages 201–202). Ask them to close their eyes and think about how they are feeling now. Ask them to silently be thankful for something in their life: perhaps their homes, families, or pets. Conclude as always with "Namaste, the light within me honors the light within you."

Time: Five to Ten Minutes

8.

The Universe and Beyond

Four- to Six-Year-Olds

Educational Elements: Freedom of movement, artistic expression, sensorial exploration, language development, sequence of activities that meets need for order

Props: Pose objects; pictures of planets and stars; yoga mats; music; construction paper; pencil, markers, crayons, or pastels; chimes; gong or singing bowl; foot lotion (optional); herbal eye pillows (optional)

Intention: Invite the children to their mats; ring your chimes, gong, or singing bowl; and welcome them to yoga. Tell them that the class will be talking about things beyond our planet, like other planets, the milky way, stars, and so on. Ask them if they knew that the sun was in fact a star, or maybe ask them if they know the names of some planets. They will have a lot to add to this discussion.

Time: Five to Ten Minutes

Warm-Up: Begin by showing the children the gateway pose from the object bag as well as the candlestick pose. Tell them to pretend that they are opening up a gateway, and then as they come into candlestick pose, have them pretend that this is how they are sitting inside a rocket ship. Tell them they are blasting off (mimic a shuttle-launch countdown) and then begin to do a little flow of poses for the rest of the warm-up.

Time: Five to Ten Minutes

Connect: Breathing rocket. Invite the children to make a "breathing rocket." They can come together to form a line (like a conga line), placing their palms on the ribs of the person in front of them, so they can feel their ribs expanding as they breath. When everyone is together, have them imagine that the rocket blasts off into space, and have them fly around the planets, stars, and meteors, moving in and out and all around. Finally, have them come apart and come in for a landing on their mats.

Time: Five to Ten Minutes

Activity: Planet journey. Tell the children they are going to now visit different planets, a few meteors, and even the sun. Show them picture cards for all these things and name them. Then place the cards on the floor all around the room. Put on some fast music and have the children run around the room, pretending that they are floating or gliding. When you stop the music, they can come in for a landing beside a card that they choose and do any yoga pose they would like or one that you demonstrate for them. Start the music again and have the children fly on, visiting many planets or stars.

Time: Approx. Ten Minutes

Breath: Darth Vader. Show the children "Darth Vader" breathing. Have them sit on their mats comfortably and close their mouths. Ask them to then place their tongues on the roof of their mouths and breathe in and out of their noses. As they exhale they should begin to make a little noise within their throats, like the sound of Darth Vader breathing. Tell them that this is a breath that will make them really warm and energized.

Time: Five Minutes

Arts and Crafts: Upside-down pictures. Set up construction paper taped to the undersides of chairs, desks, or tables, one sheet for each child. Have the children lie on their backs underneath their paper,

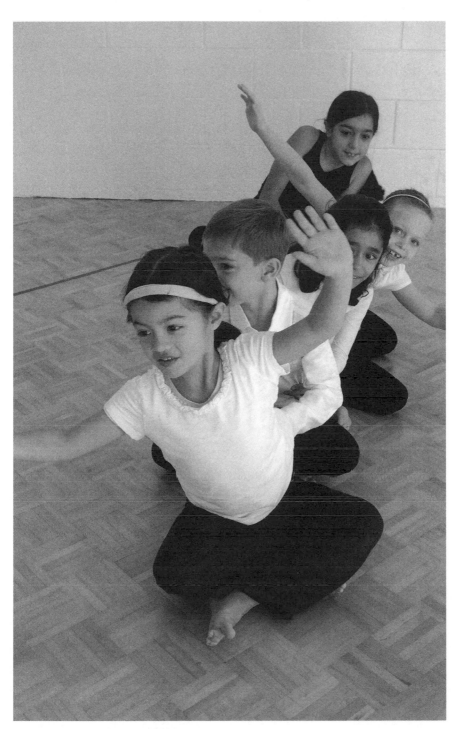

Figure 1.13. Breathing rocket

pretending they are upside down in a rocket ship. Ask them to draw whatever they think they can see from their ship. They will have lots of ideas. "Rocket Man" by Elton John is a nice song to play while the children are drawing their pictures.

Time: Ten to Fifteen Minutes

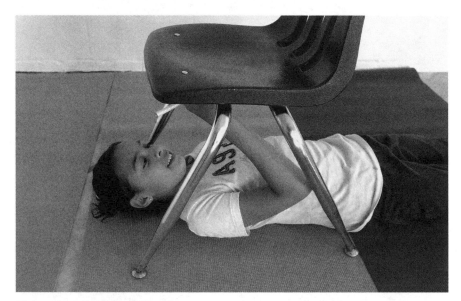

Figure 1.14. Upside-down pictures

Meditation: Signal the end of the activity and have the children return to their mats and lie down. Have them close their eyes and get comfortable. Tell them to notice how soft their breath is. Tell them that they are now weightless and are rising into space. They are going on a journey toward the end of the universe. You can point out to them all the things they will float pass (black holes, stars, galaxies, etc.) on their way. When they reach the end of the universe, they will see nothing but darkness. Now have them look back to Earth and gradually return home. Have them come in for a landing, gliding down into the atmosphere, through the clouds and toward their homes, landing in their mats.

Time: Eight to Ten Minutes

9.
Going to the Park

Four- to Six-Year-Olds

Educational Elements: Coordination, sensorial exploration, cooperation, artistic expression, development of language (names of creatures seen), balance, grace and courtesy toward each other on the trip and toward nature, freedom of choice to either observe or participate, planning and organization

Props: Animal bag filled with toy animals appropriate for going to the park (e.g., snake, fish, dog, cat, and various birds), yoga mats, herbal eye pillows, construction paper, markers or pencils, tape, appropriate music

Intention: Come together in a circle and discuss the intention for the class. For this class, the intention will be to take a trip to the park and to be aware and respectful of the natural world. The children will plan how to get there, will decide what to bring, and will discuss what they might see and how they can enjoy nature while respecting it.

Time: Five to Ten Minutes

Warm-Up: Have the children lie on their mats, pretending to sleep, then play music to wake them and have them greet the day (e.g., "Here Comes the Sun" by the Beatles). They will mirror your flow of poses. Incorporate stretching and sun salutations, and then pretend to get dressed. Have them shake out stiff spots in their body, shaking as if they are made of Jell-O. Create a little flow that lasts for the whole length of your song.

Time: Four to Five Minutes

Connect: Traffic jam. Tell the children that they are getting in their cars (if this is what they chose to travel in). Have them sit on their mats with their legs out in front—have them pretend to get in the cars, buckle up seatbelts, start engines, and drive toward the center of the circle. Have them come together (by shuffling their hips) and join feet in the middle of the circle. Ask them how they can get out of this traffic jam. Have them honk their horns. Then they should all back up to their mats. They finally arrive at the park, park their cars, and get out.

Time: Approx. Five Minutes

Activity: Park adventure. Begin by placing a hula hoop for each child in the middle of the room. Place an animal from the animal bag in the center of each hoop. Have the class join together to form the train at the park. Form a conga line with each child holding onto the next child's ribs (use music like "Locomotion" by Kylie Minogue for this). Have the children move through the park (around the hula hoops) in this train line and have them stop when you pause the music. Invite them at each stop to run to a hoop and do the pose for the animal that they find within that hoop. Allow time here for them to perfect their pose and to help them if needed. Then tell them to hop aboard the train and continue on with the music. Repeat this five or six times, asking them each time the music stops to visit a new hoop so they will do a variety of poses. When you feel that this is enough, stop the music and ask them to return to their own mats, as it is time to leave the park. Have them find their cars, start them up, and maneuver out of the parking lot. Have them park their cars at their homes—here their mats—and sit.

Time: Approx. Ten to Fifteen Minutes

Breath: Straw-sipping breath. Have them perform a cooling breath, pretending that they are drinking lemonade. Have them discuss animals they saw at the park, what the weather was like, what kind of trees they saw, and so on. The children will have lots to say.

Time: Approx. Five Minutes

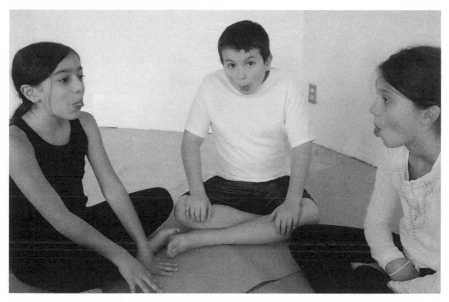

Figure 1.15. Straw-sipping breath

Arts and Crafts: Toe pictures. Tape construction paper to the walls (twelve children = twelve sheets of paper with several inches between each sheet). Have the paper just a foot or so above the ground. Have a supply of markers or colored pencils readily available. Ask the children to draw what they saw at the park today but give things a bit

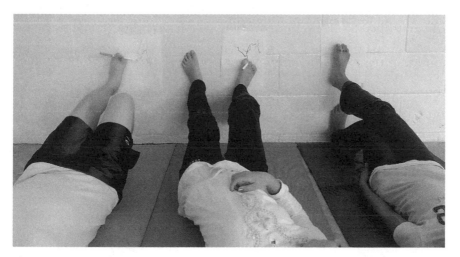

Figure 1.16. Toe pictures

of a twist by asking them to lie on their backs, place the markers in between their toes, and draw with their feet. They will love this. Some might use their hands to draw instead. Encourage discussion as they recreate their experiences on paper. A good song to play at this time is "Fireflies" by Owl City.

Time: Approx. Ten Minutes

Meditation: Have the children return to their mats. Lower the lights and hand out herbal eye pillows, should they like to place them on their eyes. Those who do not want these will let you know. Tell them to lie on their backs and let their bodies relax and melt into their mats just like butter on toast. Tell them that their bodies have become light as air and they are now floating over the park on their magic carpets, looking down on what they have experienced that day. Have them visualize what they saw at the park and imagine that the objects are so real that they can reach out and touch them. Play relaxing music (e.g., "You're Beautiful" by James Blunt). Tell them that this is their time to be still and enjoy doing absolutely nothing.

Time: Approx. Five Minutes

Gratitude: Bring the kids out of this meditation gradually by inviting them to wiggle just a few fingers, then a few toes, then one arm, then one leg, and so on. Have them bring their knees into their chests and give themselves a big hug, roll over onto one side, and finally sit up cross-legged. Have them bring their hands into a mudra (e.g., hands to their hearts). Explain how they can be thankful for this experience that they have shared with their friends, this great experience of yoga. Invite them to repeat the phrase "Namaste, the light in me honors and bows down to the light in you." End the class quietly and peacefully.

Time: Five to Ten Minutes

10.

Our Earth

Four- to Six-Year-Olds

Educational Elements: Exploring Earth's formations sensorially, language enrichment, freedom of movement, logical sequence of activities fulfilling need for order, artistic expression

Props: Blue and green scarves, blue and green modeling clay, small cardboard jewelry box lids (optional), pictures of various land and water forms, a globe, a blow-up plastic globe (optional), balloons, music, yoga mats, chimes, foot lotion (optional), herbal eye pillows (optional)

Intention: Gather the children in the usual way and welcome them to yoga. Initiate a conversation about Earth. Mention that Earth is made up of two-thirds water and only one-third land. Have a globe available so they can examine it, and ask them to show you where land is and where water is. They might show you the piece of land where they live. Encourage the discussion.

Time: Five to Ten Minutes

Warm-Up: Invite the children to do some poses for animals that live in water. They will tell you some, like fish, alligator, or frog. Then ask them to do a few poses that can be done on land. They may suggest dog, cat, or cow. Do a little flow using these poses together.

Time: Five to Ten Minutes

Connect: Pass the earth. Bring the children to the circle. Bring out a plastic, blow-up globe if you can find one or just use a balloon. Tell the children that the balloon is Earth and that every person has to work together to keep it up. Pass it around the circle—the children can only use their feet or elbows to pass it along, and the balloon can never touch the ground. Add in your own variations of how to pass the earth.

Time: Five to Ten Minutes

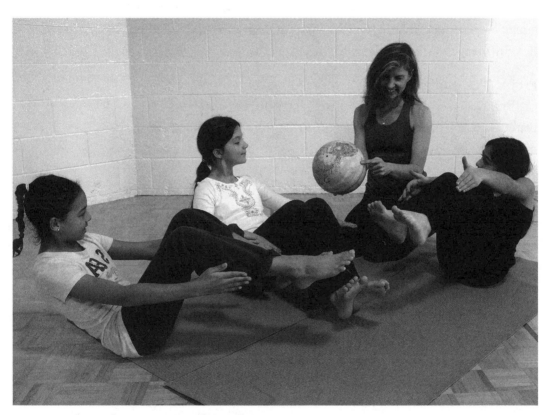

Figure 1.17. Pass the earth

Activity: Land and water forms. Tell the children that for this game, some of them are going to be the land and some of them are going to be the water. Hand out blue scarves to the children who will be water and green to those who will be land. They can switch their roles later. Tell them that the land is still and the water can begin to flow all around the land. It can move slowly or quickly, depending on the weather. The children who are the land can practice a balance in their spot if they want to. The children should practice this for a few minutes. Then bring out a card that shows a drawing of an island. Tell the children that they are going to make this. Instruct all the land children to come together to form the island and all the water children to flow around them. Tell them that an island is a body of land surrounded on all sides by water. You can then show them a picture of a lake, and they can all make it with their bodies. Continue showing them pictures of different bodies of water, such as a bay, a cape, a strait, an isthmus, a gulf, and a peninsula. They will love replicating all of these with their bodies. Then the children can switch roles and do this again.

Time: Approx. Fifteen Minutes

Arts and Crafts: Terra forms. Invite the children to make a few of the land and water forms that they learned about today. Spread your picture cards of these so the children can see them. Using green and blue modeling clay, the children can build these bodies of land and water. An option is to give out little cardboard lids from things like jewelry boxes, and the children can, for example, fill the lid with blue modeling clay and place a round green piece on top to make an island. The children can pick a few of their favorite land and water forms to make and keep.

Time: Ten to Fifteen Minutes

Partner Pose: Row the boat. Introduce the children to "row your boat" pose, pairing them up for this (refer to partner pose 3, page 189).

Time: Approx. Five Minutes

Meditation: Ring the chimes, bowl, or gong and have the children settle comfortably on their mats for their final relaxation. Offer an herbal eye pillow. Dim the lights and turn on very soft music. Tell the children to sink into their mats and breathe softly. They are now riding on a balloon that is travelling over the world. They rise up, feeling weightless. They glide next to the birds and over trees and buildings. The balloon rises up and through the clouds and then above them. Tell them they feel the sun shining down, warming them up. They see rain falling way in the distance. They look down and see land, oceans, islands, and lakes. Continue on adding your own elements to the children's balloon voyage.

Time: Eight to Ten Minutes

11.
The Holiday Season

Four- to Six-Year-Olds

Educational Elements: Grace and courtesy, cooperation, sensorial exploration, language development, freedom of movement, fulfillment of need for order

Props: Various colored pipe cleaners cut into small, medium, and large lengths; dice; pose objects bag; yoga mats; gong, chimes, or singing bowl; music; book (*Little Robin's Christmas Vest* by Jan Fearnley); foot lotion (peppermint is nice for the holidays); herbal eye pillows (optional)

Intention: Welcome the children to yoga and have them relax on their mats. Begin a discussion with them about the holiday season. You can talk about Christmas, Hanukkah, Kwanza, and any other celebrations they bring up. Ask them why does humanity celebrate these things and talk about goodwill toward other people. Tell them the intention today is to bring goodwill to others.

Time: Five to Ten Minutes

Warm-Up: Incorporate perhaps a few new poses from the pose object bag into a little vinyasa flow with the children. Demonstrate the new poses first and add them into your flow.

Time: Five to Ten Minutes

Connect: Trim the tree. Have the children seated in a circle. Have a little plastic Christmas tree in front of you and a bag of ornaments. You can use another object to hang the ornaments on if you like. Tell the children that they all must work together to decorate this tree. Hand the first ornament to the first child, perhaps using your feet to hold it. They pass it around the circle in this way until it comes back to you. You then place it on the tree. Send the next ornament around the circle, perhaps holding it between your ankles this time, and so on. After all the objects are passed, you will all have decorated the tree.

Time: Approx. Ten Minutes

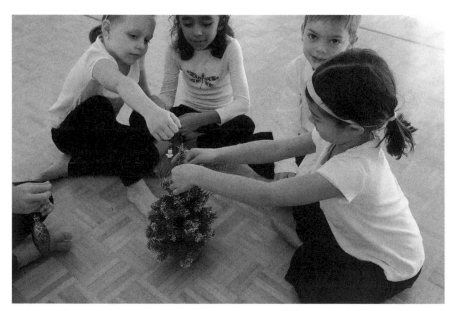

Figure 1.18. Trim the tree

Activity: Roll the dice. Bring out one dice and throw it. Tell the children that you are going to give them however many poses you roll. If it shows up as three, choose three poses you like and do them. Then pass the dice on to the next child, who then takes a turn. The other children can repeat each child's flow of poses if they like as they go.

Time: Approx. Ten Minutes

Breath: The giving breath. Tell the children that in the spirit of giving, which is what the holidays are all about, they are going to practice something called the "giving breath." Have them sit cross-legged with straight backs. Demonstrate how to do this breath: Begin with your palms turned up resting on your knees. As you inhale, raise one palm up to chest level, and as you exhale, bring it in to your heart. Inhale that hand away from you, still at chest level, and then as you exhale, place it back on your knee. Follow the same sequence now, with your other hand. Have the children mirror you for a minute or so. Discuss afterward with the children how it seemed as if they were scooping up goodness and energy and giving it to their hearts as they did the breath. This is a very grounding, calming breath exercise.

Time: Approx. Five Minutes

Arts and Crafts: Holiday snowflakes. Using precut silver, white, red, and green pipe cleaners (or whatever colors you choose), have the children make their own holiday snowflakes. Have one made already that you can show the kids. They might need help winding the pipe

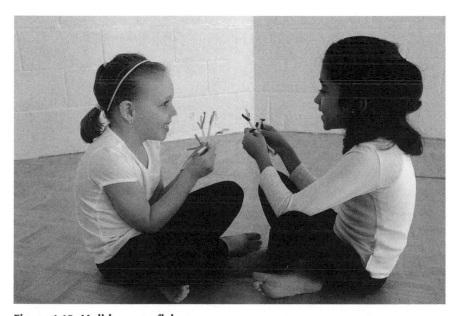

Figure 1.19. Holiday snowflakes

cleaners around each other, and the older kids can help the younger ones. When they are made, the children can move around the room with them, pretending that they are snowflakes falling to the ground.

Time: Ten to Fifteen Minutes

Book: *Little Robin's Christmas Vest* by Jan Fearnley is a wonderful holiday story that truly emphasizes the spirit of giving. Discuss it with the children afterward.

Time: Approx. Ten Minutes

Meditation: Invite the children to lie on their mats as you dim the lights for their final relaxation. As they close their eyes, tell them to notice their breath and to make it soft and even, to think about their bellies rising as they inhale and falling as they exhale. Now begin to tell a story of spreading peace around the world. You might say, "Pretend that the energy inside of your heart is spreading out now; it is a beautiful white light, reaching out to a child who lives very far away. This child needs your energy very much. That child then sends the energy on to someone else in the world, who receives it. It goes on from that child to another child somewhere else and fills them with light and goodness. Finally, all the children in our world become connected."

Time: Eight to Ten Minutes

12.
Amazing Flowers

Four- to Six-Year-Olds

Educational Elements: Attention to care of the environment, sensorial exploration, language development, freedom of movement, artistic expression

Props: Modeling clay for making flowers; yoga mats; music; foot lotion (optional); Hawaiian lei; chimes, gong, or singing bowl; pictures of flowers for children to look at during beginning group chat

Intention: Have the children relax on their mats. Ring chimes to begin the class. Welcome them to yoga. Bring out a few real flowers and show them to the group. Name them and discuss how beautiful they are. Emphasize how they make Earth smell good, how they provide food for bees, and that they should appreciate them. Engage the children in further conversation about this. Tell them that in this class they will learn more about flowers.

Time: Five to Ten Minutes

Warm-Up: If you haven't already done so, introduce the lotus pose today as well as the Venus flytrap. Demonstrate the poses and have the kids practice them. Then have the children pretend that they are little seeds. Ask them to image themselves as tiny seeds at first, gradually growing until they burst through the ground and grow tall, reaching their arms out as they open up their petals. Continue on with a vinyasa flow from this standing position.

Time: Five to Ten Minutes

Connect: Hawaiian leis. Bring out a Hawaiian lei and show it to the group. Discuss what a lei is used for and where it comes from. Tell them that it is worn around necks. Have the children pass it around the circle without using their hands—from neck to neck. After the kids have had fun with this, put the lei to the side and invite them to sit on their mats. Tell them that they are going to create a human lotus flower. Have them sit with their legs out on the mat in a V shape. Everyone should try to connect his or her feet to the next person's, and everyone should try to hold hands. Once connected, ask the kids to try to raise their feet up while still connected to their neighbor's feet, as if they were the petals of a lotus, rising up to the sky. Tell them they need to rely on the person beside them to help them balance. Make a huge rising lotus together.

Time: Approx. Ten Minutes

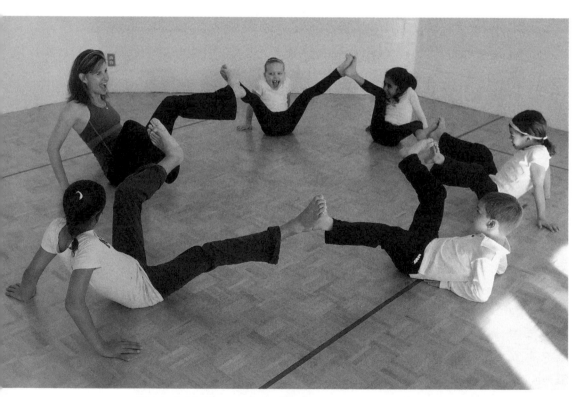

Figure 1.20. Human lotus flower

Activity: Remember your partner. Have the children spread out around the room. Invite them to play the "Remember Your Partner" game. Ask them to dance and move around when they hear the music come on. When the music stops, they need to find the person closest to them and together do one of the partner poses they just learned. The children should do three partner poses with a different child each time. When the music stops the next time, ask the children to find the person they did a certain pose with, for example, the row your boat pose, and do it again. Continue on until the children have revisited all their old partners. This is a fun memory test.

Time: Ten to Fifteen Minutes

Arts and Crafts: Lotus flowers. Have the children sit and relax. Tell them you have a story for them about the lotus flower. Have a picture of a lotus to show them. Tell them that in the world of yoga, the lotus flower is very important because it represents the journey that we all go through as human beings in life. The lotus starts its life off way down at the bottom of the pond that is very dark and muddy. The lotus has to try very hard to grow and journey to the surface of

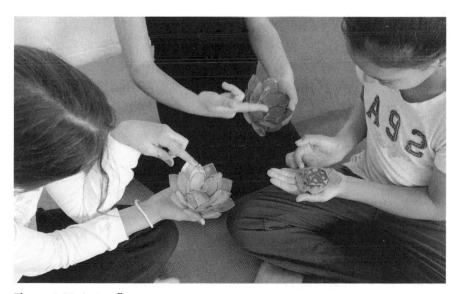

Figure 1.21. Lotus flowers

the water, and it takes a very long time. Finally, if the lotus tries hard, it emerges above the surface, with the sun shining down upon it. It opens its petals up and completes its journey. Everyone have a similar journey in life.

Then invite the children to make their own lotus flowers. Use different colored modeling clay for the petals and green modeling clay for the undersurface. Have a lotus already made as an example for the children.

Time: Ten to Fifteen Minutes

Partner Pose: Partner tree. Choose a child to demonstrate the tree pose. Have the children pair off and try the pose themselves (refer to partner pose 9, page 191).

Time: Approx. Five Minutes

Meditation: Invite the children to lie on their mats. Ring the chimes and dim the lights. Ask them to notice how their breath is soft and slow and their bodies are still. Tell them that they are now lotus flowers sinking into lily pads and feeling soft all over. They are going on a journey around a beautiful garden to look at all the other flowers. First they see a big red rose with shiny dark green leaves. Then they move on to see a daisy with white petals and a soft yellow middle. Continue with this story, including different flowers for the children to experience. Allow for some silence, and then ring the chimes.

Time: Five to Ten Minutes

Gratitude: Invite the children to slowly stretch, roll from side to side, and then sit up cross-legged. Ask them to notice how they feel inside and to close their eyes. After a moment or two, ask them to silently be grateful for all the beauty that they see around them in the natural world every day and to cherish it. End with "Namaste, the light within me honors the light within you." Bow.

Time: Five to Ten Minutes

13.
Mysteries

Four- to Six-Year-Olds

Educational Elements: Sensorial exploration, language enrichment, freedom of movement, coordination and refinement of movement, cooperation

Props: Chimes, gong, or singing bowl; items for pasting activity (e.g., sponges, cotton balls, coins, keys, wax); a cloth blindfold for each child; pose object bag; a long rope; yoga mats; foot lotion (optional); herbal eye pillows (optional); music

Intention: When the children settle to their mats, welcome them to yoga. Tell them that today they will be presented with some mysterious things that they will have to figure out. Tell them they won't be using their eyes today to solve the mysteries, so they must trust their other senses, like their sense of touch. They will also have to trust and rely on each other today.

Time: Five to Ten Minutes

Warm-Up: Invite the children to warm up. They can start by coming into a table position by placing their hands and knees on their mats at shoulder width apart. Complete the warm-up by doing a vinyasa, including poses that they are familiar with.

Time: Five to Ten Minutes

Connect: "Trust me" walk. Bring out a blindfold for each child and a long rope. Tell them that they are going to connect together—they will go for a walk blindfolded while holding the rope. Help them put on the blindfolds, and have them stand in a line holding the rope. Tell them to begin to walk, but they will have to work together to stay connected. Tell them to imagine they are stepping over a big puddle, climbing up a big hill, or jumping over a river. Ask them to notice various smells on their path like flowers or pine trees. Ask them what they can smell. Have them walk around the room. Anyone who doesn't like the blindfold can just close his or her eyes. When they return to the circle, ask them to talk about what they did on their walk and how it felt to be blindfolded.

Time: Approx. Ten Minutes

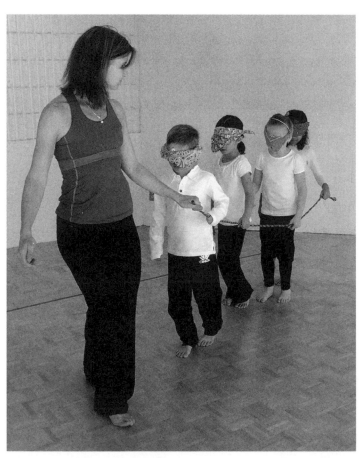

Figure 1.22. "Trust me" walk

Activity 1: Mystery objects. Invite the children to pair up with a friend. Tell them that one of them will be the leader first. The other child will be blindfolded. Give the leader four or five items that the blindfolded child can hold and try to identify (e.g., a coin, a key, an eraser, a cotton ball). When they are finished guessing, they can switch roles. Give the new leader some new items (e.g., soap, a shell, a leaf, or a pencil) so the second child can have fun guessing.

Time: Approx. Ten Minutes

Activity 2: Bat Bat, Bug Bug. Invite the children to play "Bat Bat, Bug Bug." Discuss how bats use their sense of hearing rather than their eyesight to identify their prey (echolocation). One child can be in the middle of the circle, blindfolded. He is the bat. Choose two or three children to be bugs. The rest of the children join hands and encircle them to form the "sky." The bat must find the bugs now and tag them using his sense of hearing. He says, "Bat bat," and the bugs move around within the circle answering him each time he speaks with "Bug bug." They must reply every time he speaks. If the bat walks into the children in the outer circle, they can whisper, "Sky," so he can redirect himself. When the bat has caught all the bugs, the game is over. Choose new bats and bugs and try the game again.

Time: Ten to Fifteen Minutes

Arts and Crafts: Mystery boards. The children can create their own mystery boards. They can fasten some of the items they used in the mystery objects game (activity 1) to construction paper, using a glue stick. They can then take their completed work home and play it with their family. Give them four or five items to glue to their paper.

Time: Ten to Fifteen Minutes

Partner Pose: Table and chair. Introduce the children to the table and chair pose. Have one child be the chair and another child be the table. The chair child should tuck himself into the table child. Have the children reverse their roles (refer to partner pose 5, page 190).

Time: Five to Ten Minutes

Meditation: Gather the children on their mats for a final relaxation. Have them lie down and close their eyes. Dim the lights and put on soft music. Tell them to be still and imagine that they are melting into the mat. Tell them they are exploring a wooded forest. It smells like springtime, and the birds are chirping. Tell them they feel the twigs cracking under their feet. They touch the dewy leaves. They listen to creatures making little animal noises. Ask them if they see any of these animals. Are they hiding behind trees? Maybe there is a rabbit in a hole or in a log. Tell them to smell the fresh air in the forest.

Continue with this story, and then invite the children to leave the forest and come back to their own spot, right there in the room on their mat.

Time: Eight to Ten Minutes

Gratitude: The children can begin to stretch and move, rolling over slowly and coming up to a seated position. They can place their hands in a new mudra (refer to mudras, pages 201–202).

Ask them to close their eyes and notice how they feel. Ask them to be grateful for their eyes, which allow them to see; their nose, which allows them to smell; their tongues, which allow them to taste; their ears, which let them hear, and finally their fingers, which allow them to touch. This is how they experience the world. End with "Namaste, the light in me honors the light within you." Bow to each other.

Time: Five to Ten Minutes

14.

The Skeleton

Four- to Six-Year-Olds

Educational Elements: Learning concepts of anatomy through sensorial exploration; movement; language and artistic expression; development of grace, courtesy, and cooperation

Props: Plastic skeleton that comes apart, a spine made of small wooden spools for thread, yoga mats, music, foot lotion (optional), herbal eye pillows (optional), large roll of paper for children to trace their bodies, markers or colored pencils

Intention: Direct the children to their mats and welcome them to yoga. Tell them that for this class, they are going to imagine what a blob creature looks like. The children will love this. Ask them what that blob creature would need inside of it to make it more like them, to make it be able to do yoga. Tell them that it would need bones to give it a shape. Then pass around a "spine" that you have made out of wooden empty spools of thread. To create this "spine," take five or so empty thread spools and pass an elastic through their centers. Tie a knot at each end to hold it together tightly. Explain that this spine is part of their bodies that keeps them from falling apart like goo. The kids can pass the spine around and see how it bends. Talk a bit more about bones, noting that we have 206 of them in our body. Also mention that bones are living tissue and we have many types of bones in our bodies that are long, short, flat, and irregular.

Time: Eight to Ten Minutes

Warm-Up: Begin the warm-up with the children standing. Have them shake as if they were Jell-O inside a mold. Tell them their skulls are like a mold for their brains and are a very important part of their skeleton. Introduce a few new poses from the pose bag that the children may not have seen before. Do a short flow of poses.

Time: Five to Ten Minutes

Connect 1: Shake your partner loose. Have the children choose a partner. Tell them that they have to shake their partners as if they have no bones inside them at all. One child stands over his partner, who lies on the mat. The child picks up the partner's arm and gives it a gentle little shake. The partner on the mat tries to make his arm as loose as possible so it will shake like Jell-O. Then the standing child lays their partner's arm down and lifts the next arm, jiggling it as well. Then the legs are done, one at a time. There will be uproarious laughter during this activity. After this, the children can connect together, seated in a circle. Sitting upright, the child can jiggle and shake the arm of the child to his right, while his own left arm is jiggled by the child to his left. Tell the children that they have now made a giant blob creature!

Time: Approx. Ten Minutes

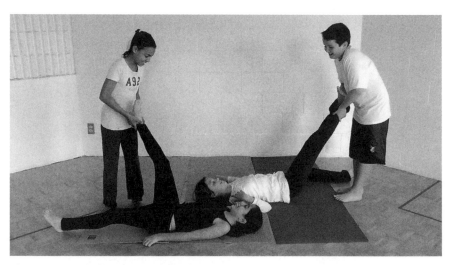

Figure 1.23. Shake your partner loose

Connect 2: Build the skeleton. Now tell the children that they have to work together again to put a skeleton together. Have a disassembled plastic skeleton and give one bone to each child. Name the bones as you hand them out. Now tell the children that you need the skull, and the child that has it places it in the middle. Then ask for the next part, the rib cage, then the pelvic bone, and so on, having each child help build the skeleton.

Time: Approx. Fifteen Minutes

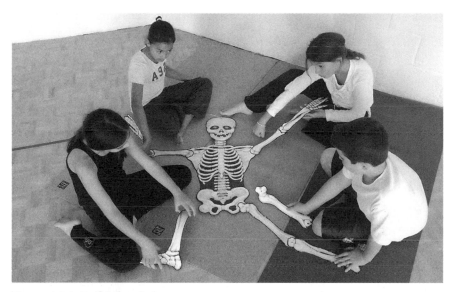

Figure 1.24. Build the skeleton

Activity: Simon says. Tell the children that you are now going to play a game using all the names of the bones from a skeleton. Start off with a simple game of Simon Says, for example, "Touch your patella" or "Touch your phalanges." If the children are comfortable with this, you can add in music for them to dance to. When the music shuts off, you can give them a direction, for example, "Place your phalanges on your rib cage," or "Place your phalanges on your tibia."

Time: Ten to Fifteen Minutes

Arts and Crafts: Drawing your body. For this craft you will need a large roll of paper that can be obtained at an art supply store. Lay out one large sheet of paper for each pair of children on the floor. Partner up the children and have one child lie on the paper and have the other child trace around their friend's body with a marker. The younger children may just want to trace their torso. Display the plastic skeleton that you made earlier for the children to use as a model. They can then draw that skeleton or some of their bones on the inside of their traced body pictures. They can color them if they wish. Remember to keep reinforcing the names of the bones to the children.

Time: Approx. Fifteen Minutes

Book: If time allows, read *Dem Bones* by Bob Barner.

Time: Five to Ten Minutes

Meditation: Invite the children to lie on their mats for their final relaxation. Dim the lights and have them close their eyes and breathe softly. Tell them to soften their bodies and sink into their mats. Begin by saying, "Notice your toes now, and feel how they tingle. Now let's move on to your feet—notice just your feet and feel them." Then move on to their ankles, legs, hips, bellies, and so on, until you have done a full body scan. Do this very slowly, mentioning the names of some of the bones you have talked about in the class. Finally end up at the tip of their skulls, and then ask them to relax their entire bodies.

Time: Eight to Ten Minutes

Gratitude: Ask the children to stretch now, roll over slowly, and come to a seated position. Ask them to close their eyes and silently be grateful for their strong bodies and strong bones. Ask them to be grateful for their good health and their ability to exercise to stay fit. End with "Namaste, the light inside of me honors the light inside of you." Bow to each other.

Time: Five to Ten Minutes

15.
Sounds and Words

Four- to Six-Year-Olds

Educational Elements: Language enrichment through sensorial exploration and movement, grace and courtesy, cooperation, self-care

Props: A collection of cardboard letters, including the most commonly used ones for making simple words; book (*A Is for . . . ?: A Photographer's Alphabet* by Henry Hounstein); yoga mats; music; foot lotion (optional); chimes, singing bowl, or gong; herbal eye pillows (optional)

Intention: Invite the children to be seated on their mats and welcome them to yoga. Talk about how you know they all love books and they are learning how to read all the wonderful words inside books. Talk about how all words are made up of letters and how all letters make sounds. Ask them to tell you some letters and some sounds. Tell them that they are going to do some yoga with these letters and sounds.

Time: Five to Ten Minutes

Warm-Up: Ask the children if they can make a few letters with their bodies. Try *C* and *O* to start off with. The children will have lots of ideas. Give them each a little turn. Then do a little vinyasa flow for them to follow.

Time: Eight to Ten Minutes

Connect: Word connect. Tell the children you are going to play a word connect game. They need to work together to create words. Give them each a little cardboard letter to hold onto. Each child gets a different letter. Call out a word, like "cat." Ask them what the first sound in "cat" is. The child holding C will bring it forward. Ask them what the next sound in cat is. The child with the A will come forward. Finally, the child with the T will come forward. They can spell the word out on the floor. Now give them a new word, like "dog" or "bird," making sure everyone gets a turn to spell a word. The older children will help the younger children a lot with this game.

Time: Ten to Fifteen Minutes

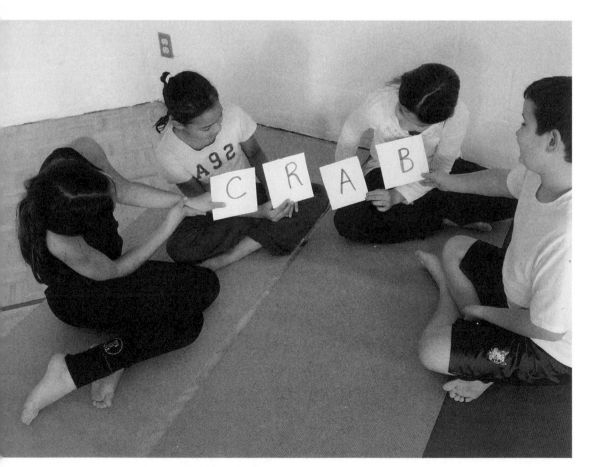

Figure 1.25. Word connect

Activity: P is for pose. Put on some fun music, and the children can begin to dance however they like in the room. Turn off the music and call out a letter, for example, *A*. Ask them, "What pose can we do that starts with the letter *A*"? The children might call out the word "alligator" and may do its pose, remembering it from the pose object bag. Or they may invent their own new pose, like "apple," and may make that shape with their body. Let the children enjoy the freedom of making up poses as you continue this game. After calling out several letters, have the children finally return to their mats.

Time: Ten to Fifteen Minutes

Book: *A Is for. . .?: A Photographer's Alphabet* by Henry Hounstein

Time: Approx. Ten Minutes

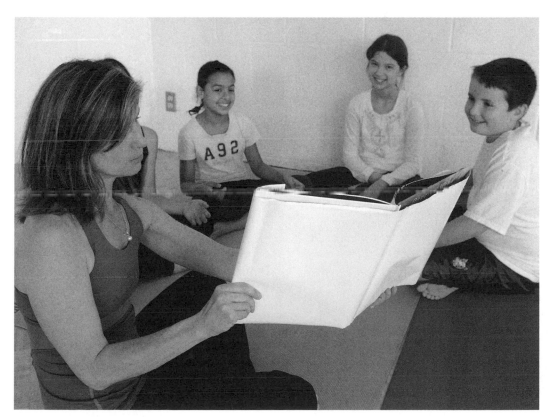

Figure 1.26. Reading the book

Partner Pose: Lizard on a rock. Introduce the children to the lizard on a rock pose. Tell them that the lizards are basking in the sun. One child is the rock and the other is the lizard (refer to partner pose 6, page 190).

Time: Five to Ten Minutes

Meditation: When the children are lying on their mats, relaxed with their eyes closed, dim the lights and put on soft music. Tell them that they are going to glide on their mats through a zoo. This is a special zoo; it is the "Alphabet Zoo." As they enter the zoo, the first cage has an alligator in it, very green and scaly. They then come to the bear, very furry and brown. In their journey, they pass the cobra, the dolphin, the elephant, and so on. Guide the children through the zoo, asking them to imagine what the animals look like. Then tell them it is time to leave and glide back to their homes and into their beds after their long day at the zoo. Ring the chimes softly.

Time: Ten Minutes

Gratitude: Ask the children to gradually roll over and come up to a seated position with their eyes closed. Ask them to pause for a minute and notice how they feel. Ask them to be silently thankful for their time together today and for all the things they are able to learn from reading stories and books. Ask them to be thankful that they are learning to read, and through reading they can learn so much. End with "Namaste, the light in me honors the light within you." Bow to each other.

Time: Five to Ten Minutes

16.
Shapes and Numbers

Four- to Six-Year-Olds

Educational Elements: Sequence of the class caters to child's need for order, freedom of movement, sensorial exploration of concepts of numbers and shapes, language enrichment

Props: Stamps or markers for children to make poses with, precut paper shapes (triangles, squares, pentagons, etc.), music, yoga mats

Intention: Gather the children and welcome them to yoga. Explain that today they will talk about shapes and numbers. Ask them if they can name some, and as you discuss them, ask them to tell you how many sides the shape they are naming has. Tell them that numbers will be important in this class as well.

Time: Five to Ten Minutes

Warm-Up: Pair the children. Assign a number to each pair. Have each pair of children lie of the floor and try to create their number with their bodies.

Time: Five to Ten Minutes

Connect 1: Pass the squeeze. Join hands together in a circle. Ask the children to help each other allow your squeeze of energy to travel all around and get back to you. Squeeze the child's hand to your right, and he or she in turn squeezes the person to his or her right, and so on. Different children can start the squeeze off too. You can switch this game up by having the children "pass the pose." They whisper

Creative Yoga for Children

a pose to a child, and the pose continues around the circle. The last child to get it does the pose for the group. This is a little variation on the broken telephone game.

Time: Eight to Ten Minutes

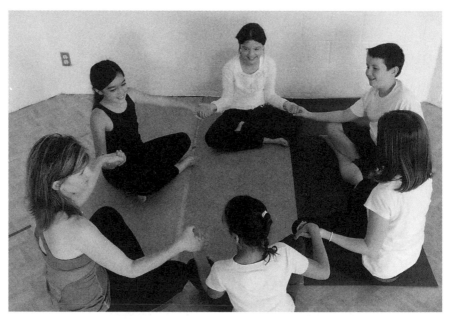

Figure 1.27. Pass the squeeze

Connect 2: The number flow. Have the children together either sitting or standing in a circle. Tell them that you are going to start a flow of poses. The first child calls out the number one and chooses one pose to do on his or her mat. The second child calls out the number two, does the first child's pose plus one of his or her own. Once you get up to the higher numbers, the children can help remind each other of the poses. This is great memory practice!

Time: Five to Ten Minutes

Connect 3: Make a shape. Tell the children that they are going to work together to make shapes with their bodies. Call on one child to make a line by lying on the floor, very straight. Then ask a second child to turn that line into an angle. They should lie near the first child, connecting either at the feet or at the head to form an angle. Then call on a third child to make the angle into a triangle. The child joins the first two, lying down and connecting to form the shape. Continue on this way creating next a square, pentagon, hexagon, and so on—remember to name the shape as you make it and have the children count the sides.

Time: Five to Ten Minutes

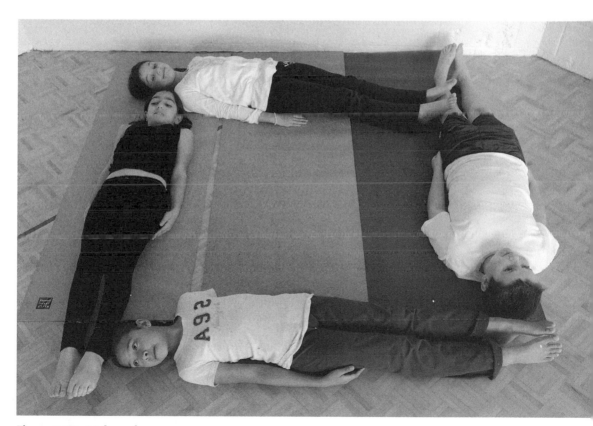

Figure 1.28. Make a shape

Activity: What's your number? Hand out a slip of paper to each child with a number written on it. Lay out a selection of pose cards. The children should then take the number of cards that their slip of paper indicates. They lay the cards out on their mats. When the children have all positioned themselves on mats around the room, ask them to leave their cards and numbers on the mats. They can then do the poses that they have. Turn on music and have them move or dance around the room. Turn off the music and ask them to choose a new mat to go to and do the number of poses that they see there. Continue on in this way until the children have visited several mats.

Time: Ten to Fifteen Minutes

Breath: Invite the children to relax and return to their mats. Ask them to do the "countdown" breath. With their mouth closed, have them inhale through their noses. Count to five, pause, and then count back down to one. Repeat this a few times to relax them, and then ask them how they are feeling.

Time: Approx. Five Minutes

Arts and Crafts: Shapes. Hand out three or four paper shapes that you have created to each child. Ask the children to write the number of sides each of their shapes have on one side of the paper and write the names of the shapes on the other side.

Time: Approx. Ten Minutes

Meditation: Dim the lights and have the children lie down. Offer them herbal eye pillows and turn on soothing music. Tell them to close their eyes, let their bodies completely sink into their mats, and breathe softly. Explain that the sun is shining warmly down on them. Tell them to feel it warming their face. Tell them to feel it on their neck, their shoulders, and all along their arms. Tell them to feel the sun on their hands and on each finger, one at a time. Now they should feel the rays of sun shining right onto their heart, making their heart open up. Now they should feel it on their chest and on their stomach. They should feel the sun moving down their legs to their knees and down to their ankles, feet, and toes. They should feel their toes tingling in the heat of the sun. Now the sun is shining brighter and it shines over their whole body. Gradually now, the sun is setting for the day. Tell them to watch it in their mind, sinking lower in the sky. They should watch how it turns different colors: yellow, orange, red, and pink. It lowers further. They can only see half of it now on top of the ground. It is getting lower, and now they can only see a glimmer of light left from it. It is finally gone for the day. Tell them to relax; it will be back tomorrow.

Time: Eight to Ten Minutes

Gratitude: Ring the chimes softly to end the meditation. Ask the children to stretch and to slowly roll over to one side, then come up to a seated position. Have them bring their hands to their hearts with their eyes closed and ask them to notice how relaxed they feel. Ask them to silently be grateful for all the things that keep them safe in their lives: police officers, firefighters, crossing guards, teachers, and their parents. Ask them to think of other people that make them feel safe. End with "Namaste, the light within me honors the light within you." Bow.

Time: Five to Ten Minutes

17.
Forest Life

Four- to Six-Year-Olds

Educational Elements: Sensorial exploration of botany and zoology, language enrichment, need for order, freedom of movement, balance and refinement of movement

Props: Yoga mats; chimes, singing bowl, or gong; pose object bag; book (*Little Beaver and the Echo* by Amy MacDonald); placemats and books to use as lily pads and river rocks (whatever you have on hand will work); music; scarves or ribbons

Intention: Welcome your class to yoga and have them sit on their mats. Tell them that they will be going into the forest on a journey. They will see different animal habitats there. Ask them if they know any mammals that live in the forest, what kind of reptiles lives there, what kinds of amphibians live there, and so on. The children will tell you all about their various hikes and adventures into forests.

Time: Five to Ten Minutes

Warm-Up: Tell the children that there often are lots of mosquitoes in the forest, and they should put on some bug spray for their journey. Have them do this, and then show them the mosquito pose, which they may not have already seen. Then lead them through a little flow, including several animal poses they may find in a forest.

Time: Five to Ten Minutes

Connect: Forest storm. Invite the children to stand together in a circle. Have half the children be a tree (they can think of a kind of tree they would like to be, like a maple or an elm), and have them go into tree pose. The other half of the children can be the wind. They can carry ribbons or scarves if they wish as they travel in and out of the trees and around the room. Tell a story about how the storm is starting in the forest, and the wind starts moving through it first softly, then quicker and quicker, causing the trees to sway back and forth. The wind grows so much that it almost topples them down. Then the trees decide to come together and support each other (the children who are trees can all join hands). Their connection has saved them. The wind cannot harm them now, and the storm dies down. Have the children switch roles.

Time: Eight to Ten Minutes

Activity: Cross the river. Invite the children to practice some of the balances they have already learned (e.g., flamingo, tree, and eagle). Then lay out a little course for them to cross, using lily pads and rocks (different colored placemats). Explain that they are going to cross the river to the green grassy bank, but in order to do so, they must travel across on the rocks and lily pads so they don't fall in the water. If they fall off, they can swim back and start the course again. The lily pads are safe, so they can stand on them and rest, but as they step on each rock, they must do a balance of their choice before hopping on to the next lily pad. The children waiting on the sides can pretend to be different river animals (e.g., fish, frog). The children can have a few turns each crossing the river.

Time: Ten to Fifteen Minutes

Breath: Wind on the pond breath. The children should sit together to form a pond, cupping their hands in their laps. Ask them to think of a thought that bothers them or something they don't feel happy about. Ask them to breathe in energy, and with every exhalation, tell them that their unhappy thought is slipping down into the pond. Finally, a big breath out will blow every negative thought that is in the pond away. Encourage the children to use this breath on their own whenever they need to. It is very soothing.

Time: Approx. Five Minutes

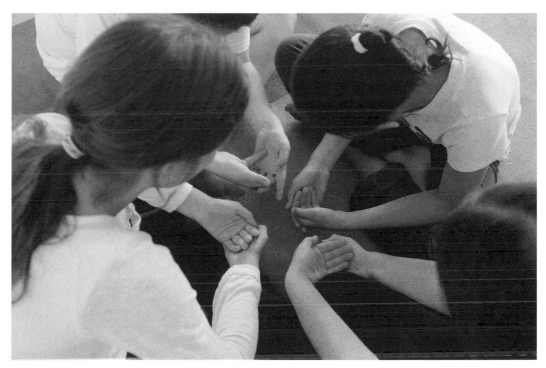

Figure 1.29. Wind on the pond breath

Book: *Little Beaver and the Echo* by Amy MacDonald. This book will revisit some of the poses that the children have been practicing during this class, and they can demonstrate them as they listen to the story.

Time: Five to Ten Minutes

Partner Pose: Twist and Turn stretch. Invite the children to sit down and partner them off for this pose (see partner pose 8, page 191). The children sit cross-legged in front of their partner with their knees touching. They each put their right hands behind their backs, and with their other hands, they grab their partner's left hand. They take a big breath, and as they breathe out, they twist away from their partner, looking over the partner's right shoulder.

Time: Five to Ten Minutes

Meditation: Ring your chimes, gong, or singing bowl and have the children relax on their mats as you dim the lights. Ask them to relax and close their eyes as you put on tranquil music. Tell them that they are sinking into their lily pads, which are warm and soft. Now they journey down the river that they crossed earlier slowly. They will see all the animals that live in the forest. The animals are all coming to the river bank to meet them. They see first the frogs in the water, jumping up and diving down. They see fish below and baby alligators peeking out of the water. Add your own elements into this little journey down the river. Include the weather, how the air feels, and so on. Finally, bring them back to the bank of the river where they can roll off their lily pad onto the warm grass.

Time: Eight to Ten Minutes

Gratitude: Ring your chimes and ask the children to slowly stretch. They can bring their knees into their chests, giving themselves a big hug. Then they can roll over and come up to a seated position. Invite them to bring their hands to a new mudra, called the Venus lock mudra (refer to page 202).

Tell them that this mudra make them feel warm and loved. Ask them to be silently grateful in their minds that they have so many clean, beautiful forests around that people all work together to sustain and keep clean. Because of this the animals can continue living there safely.

Time: Five to Ten Minutes

18.
Sniff, Touch, and Listen

Four- to Six-Year-Olds

Educational Elements: Identification of concepts through movement and sensorial exploration, language enrichment, benefit of mixed age group (older assisting younger), coordination and refinement of movement, activities that work toward instilling a sense of independence

Props: Various items that the children can readily identify the smell of (e.g., cinnamon, lemon, peppermints, and various smelling lotions), books (*The Black Book of Colors* by Menena Cottin and *My Five Senses* by Aliki), music, yoga mats, chimes, gong or singing bowl, herbal eye pillows (small scented pillows that can be purchased at yoga stores or studios), pose object bag

Intention: Invite the children to sit down on their mats. Welcome them to yoga. Tell them that they are going to use their five senses to identify things. Ask them if they know what their senses are. Have a discussion about each one of them, eliciting as much language from the children as you can.

Time: Five to Ten Minutes

Warm-Up: Invite the children to stand up on their mats. Tell them that you are going to do some laundry today. Have them pretend to load the washing machine and then turn it on. Tell them that they are the part of the machine, which twists back and forth, washing the clothes. Have them twist back and forth faster and faster, with their arms waving out to the sides. Gradually slow down and stop. Then have them pretend to unload the clothes and put them into the dryer. Have them pretend that they are the clothes swirling around in the dryer. The children can move all around or they can be in a little ball on their mats, rolling back and forth. They can move in any way that they think the clothing would. At the end of the dryer cycle, have them unload the clothes and pretend to get dressed.

Time: Five to Ten Minutes

Connect: Pose meets pose. Lay out either some pose objects or pose cards in front of you for all the children to see. Invite the first child to choose one. The child should demonstrate the pose and stay hold it. The second child should then choose a pose but must demonstrate it with one part of their body connected to some part of the first child's. They must be careful not to impede each other's balance; in

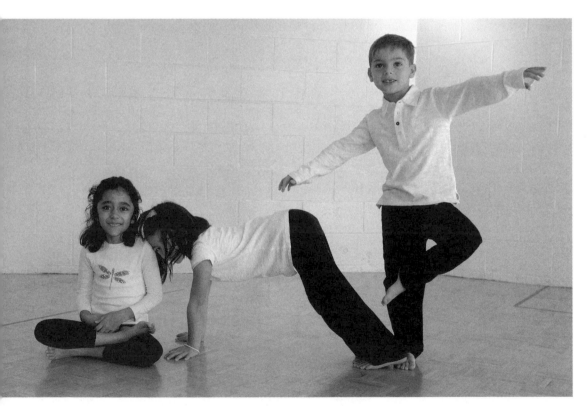

Figure 1.30. Pose meets pose

fact they can try to support the other child in some way if they can. The children continue doing their poses until they are all connected in a long line together.

Time: Eight to Ten Minutes

Activity 1: Creating a band. Ask the children to sit in a circle as quietly as they possibly can and close their eyes. Ring your chimes, and ask them to listen to the whole vibration of the sound, trying to actually feel it. When it ends tell them to notice the sound of complete silence. Wait a minute or two, and then ask the children one by one what they heard during that silence. Perhaps they heard a bird outside, a radiator humming, or a car honking on the road. Ask them to make that sound themselves. When all the children have demonstrated a sound, then ask them to make these sounds all together, creating a song!

Time: Eight to Ten Minutes

Activity 2: What's that smell? Tell the children that they are going to try to identify some smells. Partner them off, with one child blindfolded. The unblindfolded child presents three or four objects that have a particular smell to the first child, who tries to guess what each of them are. Have the "smellables" packaged in separate Ziploc bags.

Many things can be used (e.g., nutmeg, cinnamon, garlic, pepper, lemon, lime, peppermints, and various smelling creams and lotions).

Once the blindfolded child has had a turn, the children can switch places, and new objects can be presented.

Time: Ten Minutes

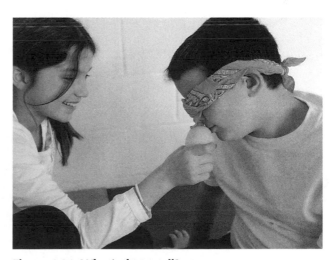

Figure 1.31. What's that smell?

Book: *The Black Book of Colors* by Menena Cottin. Every page of this book is completely black, so ask the children to imagine the colors as they hear about them. They can also touch the tactile surface of the pages.

Alternatively, *My Five Senses* by Aliki is a wonderful book about the senses for young children.

Time: Five to Ten Minutes

Meditation: Ring the chimes and invite the children to relax on their mats. Dim the lights, turn on soothing music, and have them close their eyes. If the children want herbal eye pillows, be sure to ask them to describe the smell of the eye pillow. Tell the children to get comfortable and let the world around them just slowly slip away. They are now lying in a beautiful field of flowers, gazing up at the blue sky. Ask them to notice the sweet smell that the flowers have. The first flowers they see are bright yellow buttercups. They hold them up against their skin and notice the yellow reflection that shines up against it. Then they notice bright red roses. They smell their sweet smell. Take the children on a trip around this field of flowers, naming many of them. Tell them they notice the flowers' colors and smells. Finally they feel tired and lay softly back down in the field, and their mat transports them back to their yoga class.

Time: Eight to Ten Minutes

Gratitude: Ring the chimes, and ask the children to slowly move their fingers, and then their toes. Tell them to stretch and move however they feel they need to. Then they may roll over onto one side and bring themselves to a seated position. They may bring their hands into any mudra that they would like. Ask them to silently be grateful for this day and for yoga class. They should also be grateful for their eyes that help them see everything in their world, their ears that let them hear beautiful sounds, their tongues that let them taste delicious food, their noses that let them smell flowers and fresh rain on the grass, and finally for their fingers and toes that they use to feel fuzzy fur and warm bath water. End with "Namaste, the light within me honors the light within you." Bow.

Time: Five to Ten Minutes

19.
Metamorphosis

Four- to Six-Year-Olds

Educational Elements: Freedom of choice, order, language enrichment, freedom of movement, artistic expression, refinement of the writing hand

Props: Long strips of paper (enough for each child), colored pencils, book (*Chickens Aren't the Only Ones* by Ruth Heller), music, ping-pong ball, chimes, gong or singing bowl, feathers, yoga mats

Intention: Gather the children and have them sit on their mats. Welcome them to yoga. Explain to them that they are going to talk about metamorphosis. This is when something starts out as one thing and then changes its form and turns into something new. Discuss the metamorphosis of a caterpillar into a butterfly. Ask them if they know of any other creatures that go through this process. Talk about tadpoles turning into frogs and other of the children's suggestions.

Time: Five to Ten Minutes

Warm-Up: From their bunny poses, have the children stretch up to the sky and begin with a few sun salutations. Continue with a short flow.

Time: Approx. Five Minutes

Connect: Move the egg. Have the children in a circle, seated on their mats. Bring out a ping-pong ball and explain to them that it is your egg. Ask them to carefully use their breath to blow the egg from person to person, being careful not to break it. Ask them to send it all the way around the circle and back to you. Tell them to use soft breath and try not to use their hands. They must work together to preserve the egg.

Time: Approx. Five Minutes

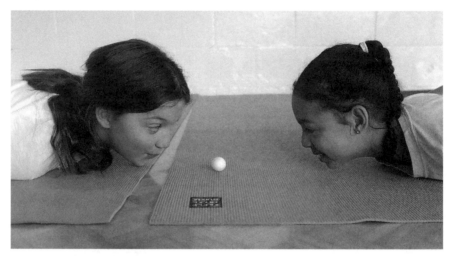

Figure 1.32. Move the egg

Activity 1: Growing up. Ask the children to do a child's pose on their mats. Tell them that they are chicks inside an egg and that they are floating and growing. Tell them that they are ready to come out of the egg and become a chick. Have them walk around like baby chicks. Then tell them that they are finally changing into grown roosters and hens. Let them move around now as full grown chickens, scratching, pecking, and having fun. They can try this again, this time as a different creature, like a lizard in its soft-shelled egg, a tadpole in its jelly egg, or even as a caterpillar larva in its cocoon. They will have suggestions of their own as well.

Time: Approx. Ten Minutes

Activity 2: Tickle time. Divide the group of children into partners. Ask half the class to be little chicks inside of their eggs, very still and small.

Tell them to close their eyes; they are sleeping. The other children should then wake them up slowly using a feather. The children tickle a part of the sleeping children's bodies (e.g., a toe, knee, or finger), and the sleeping children must identify the part of the body to their partners. Have them tickle them in four or five spots, and then switch partners. There will be uproarious laughter during this game!

Time: Approx. Five Minutes

Breath: Bunny breathing. Introduce "Bunny Breathing" to the children. Have them squat like bunnies and wrinkle their noses. Ask them to breathe in and out many times, through only their noses. After the breath exercise ask them if they feel ready to warm up.

Time: Three to Five Minutes

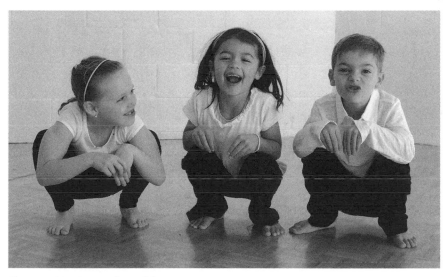

Figure 1.33. Bunny breathing

Arts and Crafts: Morphing strips. Using one long strip of paper and colored pencils, the children can draw out the metamorphosis of any creature they choose, starting on the left side with the first stage (e.g., egg) of the creature's life and finishing on the right with the developed creature. They may even want to do the growth of a seed into a tree or flower instead of an animal.

Time: Approx. Ten Minutes

Book: *Chickens Aren't the Only Ones* by Ruth Heller. The children can act out the animal poses in the book as you read through it.

Time: Five to Ten Minutes

Meditation: Using chimes, invite the children to come to their mats, lie down, close their eyes, and get nice and still. Dim the lights and turn on soft music. Ask them to breathe softly and let all their thoughts trickle out of their minds. Now ask them to begin to imagine a perfect vacation spot. Maybe it is on a beach, in the mountains, or at a park. Tell them to imagine that they are there. Imagine what the weather is like. Is it sunny, cool, or warm? Imagine that their favorite meal is now being served to them on their vacation. What is this meal? Imagine what it tastes like. Now they are looking at their favorite animals that have come along on the trip. What are they? What are their favorite items that they have packed for this trip? Carry on with this story, adding in your own elements. Finally, have the children return from their vacation to their mats, rejuvenated from their trip.

Time: Five to Ten Minutes

Gratitude: Ask the children to move their toes and fingers. Then have them stretch one arm and one leg, then the other arm and leg, and gradually roll over onto one side. Then come up into a seated position, using any mudra they would like, keeping their eyes closed. Ask them to silently be grateful for their imaginations. Their imaginations let them go anywhere in the world and do whatever they want to do. They allow them to dream about doing wonderful things without ever having to leave the room. The use of their minds is a great gift that they have. End with "Namaste, the light within me honors the light within you." Bow.

Time: Five to Ten Minutes

20.
Point of Arrival Class

Four- to Six-Year-Olds

Educational Elements: grace and courtesy, freedom of choice, freedom of movement, language enrichment, need for order, coordination, and refinement of the writing hand

Props: Yoga bingo cards; counters to put on the cards (many things can be used); pipe cleaners (various colors if possible); book (*Eggbert the Slightly Cracked Egg* by Tom Ross); music; yoga mats; gong, chimes, or singing bowl

Intention: Ring the chimes and gather the children. Welcome them to yoga, and tell them that today's class will be a celebration of all the things they have experienced in the course so far. They have done so many things, and they will be able to choose which activities they have liked most and do a few of them again. Have a short discussion about what things they may like to do. Also tell them that there will be a surprise game toward the end of the class!

Time: Five to Ten Minutes

Warm-Up: Put together a long flow, using many of the poses the children have enjoyed doing so far.

Time: Five to Ten Minutes

Connect: Children's choice. This will be the children's choice. They may want to do the pass the pose or pass the squeeze activity. A favorite may be forming a conga line and doing a Breathing Train. Let the children choose.

Time: Five to Ten Minutes

Activity 1: Allow some time now for the children to choose a group activity that they have enjoyed. A favorite may be "Bat Bat, Bug Bug," or a simple "Freeze Flow" game with you calling out different pose names. Keep this relatively short and simple.

Time: Ten to Fifteen Minutes

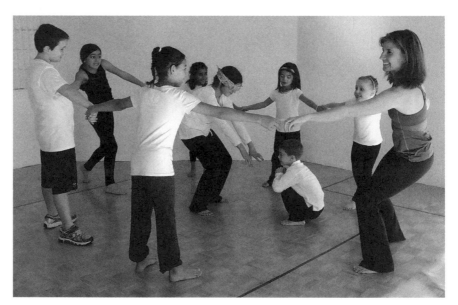

Figure 1.34. Bat Bat, Bug Bug game

Activity 2: Yoga bingo. Give out a bingo card and a handful of counters to each child. Tell them that they play this game just as they do regular bingo, but on every square of their cards, they will see a pose. Tell them that if you call out that pose, they should cover it with their counter and do the pose as well. When their whole card is covered, they may yell, "Bingo!" Pull the yoga poses out of the pose object bag, one at a time, calling them out. When one child has completed his or her card, continue calling more poses until everyone is finished. The prize will be for everyone, and it is something that they can make.

Time: Approx. Ten Minutes

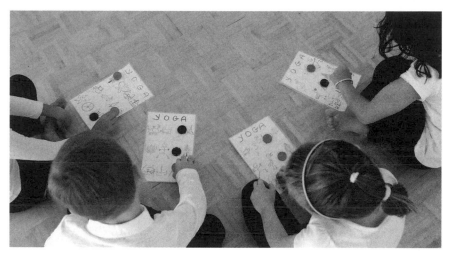

Figure 1.35. Yoga bingo

Breath: Back breathing in child's pose. Have the children come into child's pose after their warm-up. Ask them to feel the sides of their backs as they breathe. Ask them to feel how their ribs expand out sideways every time they breathe in. Have them breathe like this for a minute, noticing how their lungs and rib cages move in and out.

Time: Three to Five Minutes

Arts and Crafts: Yoga man. Hand out four short pipe cleaners to each child. Tell them that this is going to be their prize and it is a yoga person who they can put into any pose. Demonstrate how to make the head into a circle first. Connect the body to it, then twist one pipe cleaner around this center piece to make the arms. Finally, twist the last piece around the bottom of the torso to make the legs. They can have fun putting their yoga man into many poses.

Time: Approx. Ten Minutes

Book: *Eggbert the Slightly Cracked Egg* by Tom Ross. Tell the children that Eggbert represents everyone and ask them what this story teaches them.

Time: Five to Ten Minutes

Meditation: Ring the chimes for a final meditation and have the children lie down on their mats, eyes closed. Tell them to let go of their day and soften their bodies. Dim the lights and put on meditative music. Ask the children if they can concentrate just on their hearts. Ask them to listen for their heartbeat and feel it beating in their chests. Ask them to begin imagining that a little purple light is beginning to grow and shine inside their heart. The light is growing brighter. Finally, this purple light bursts through and shines out of their bodies, sending itself out toward the world. It gets bigger and bigger and shines on the whole city, making it bright and warm. Then it grows even bigger and shines out all over the country, touching everyone. The light hasn't finished growing, and finally it crosses the oceans to all the countries in the earth. The light from their hearts has travelled all over the world. They can touch everyone with light and warmth if they open their hearts and let it out. Keep imagining this purple light, glowing strong, all around the earth. Keep it going. Breathe softly. When they are ready, they can bring the light back in to their hearts, keeping it ready to go whenever they want to send it out. Tell them to relax and rest.

Time: Eight to Ten Minutes

Gratitude: Ring the chimes, and slowly bring the children out of their meditation, having them stretch and roll over onto one side. As they come into a seated position, ask them to bring their hands into any mudra they would like and to keep their eyes closed. Ask them to silently be grateful for one another. Staying connected to all their friends and other human beings is important. They should be grateful for any connection and treasure it. End with "Namaste, the light in me honors the light within you." Bow.

Time: Five to Ten Minutes

Part II:
Class Themes
Seven- to Nine-Year-Olds

1. Botany
2. Muscles
3. Fun with Words
4. Zoology
5. The Body Systems
6. Countries of the World
7. The Creation of the Universe
8. Drama/Performance
9. Shapes and Angles
10. Animal, Vegetable, or Mineral

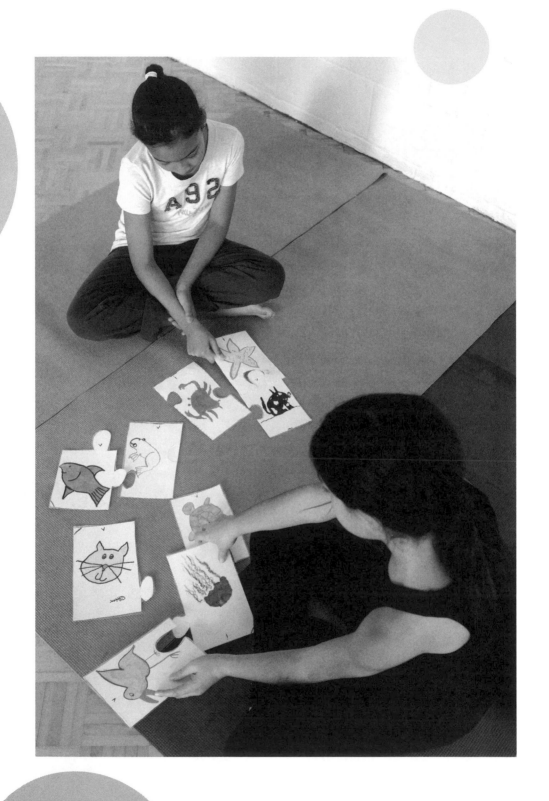

1.

Botany

Seven- to Nine-Year-Olds

Educational Elements: Language enrichment, absorbing various elements of botany in a sensorial way, freedom of movement, freedom of choice, cooperation

Props: Pictures of various carnivorous plants (e.g., Venus flytrap, pitcher, sundew), set of cards that illustrate one particular part of a plant on each (e.g., stem, corolla, roots, root hairs, calyx, leaves, stamens, pistil), modeling clay in various colors, yoga mats, music, chimes, herbal eye pillows, bag of dried beans or chick peas

Intention: Invite the children to join you on their mats, in a circle if possible. Ring the chimes, and welcome them to yoga. When they are settled, tell them that they will be discussing all kinds of plants—including strange and weird ones! Tell them that there are plants that actually eat animals. Ask them if they know of any. Explain that the sundew plant has tentacles that look like fireworks. The tentacles are sticky so that it can trap flies. The pitcher plant looks like a test tube with a lid. When insects crawl inside, the lid closes on them. Try to have pictures of these plants on hand or draw them for the children. Invite more conversation, explaining why these plants need living animals as sustenance, as their mineral supply in their soil might be low.

Time: Approx. Five to Ten Minutes

Warm-Up: Ask the children to curl up on their mats, pretending to be seeds planted in the soil. Now they slowly grow, getting taller, breaking through the earth, and blooming. Tell the children to be as big with their bodies as possible. Now begin a little flow of poses to music.

Time: Approx. Five to Ten Minutes

Connect: Parts of the flower. Display a set of cards that illustrate the seed of a flower, the root, the root hairs, the corolla, the stem, the calyx, the pistil, and the stamens. Each child will choose a card with a "part" on it (there will be some duplicates depending on the size of the group). Ask the children who have the root to come to the middle of the circle first and place their cards on the floor. Next, ask the children who have root hairs to place them on the root cards. Then have the stem card holders place their cards down, and so on. Work your way up the plant until everyone has worked together to build the flower. Have the children admire their work.

Time: Ten to Fifteen Minutes

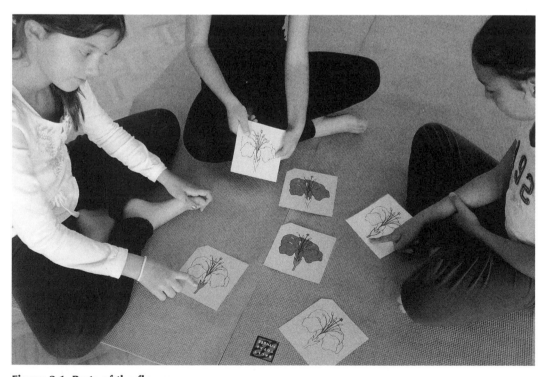

Figure 2.1. Parts of the flower

Activity: Feed the beast. Gather the children, using your chimes if you like. Explain that in this game, there will be two children who are carnivorous plants. These two children will chase the others in a game similar to tag. The other children will have one bean (you can use a dried chick pea), which will be their insect. Tell them that if they are tagged, they can feed it to the carnivorous plant in order to survive and get away, but they can only use this once—if they are tagged again they must sit out. The children can choose which carnivorous plant they would like to be each round and can have fun choosing which insect they would like their dried bean to be.

Time: Ten to Fifteen Minutes

Breath: The children will be very warm after their game, so have them sit and do a relaxing breathing exercise by curling their tongues in the shape of straws and inhaling through them. Then they can close their mouths and exhale through their noses. Do this several times.

Time: Five Minutes

Arts and Crafts: Man-eating plants. Show the children pictures of the plants you have discussed today and invite them to make a little clay model of the plant of their choice. Have a few different colors of modeling clay available.

Time: Approx. Ten Minutes

Meditation: Dim the lights and invite the children to lie down on their mats. You can give them an herbal eye pillow if they would like one. Tell them to let their arms fall down to their sides with their palms open. Have them imagine they are sinking into the earth below them, with roots growing down from them into the earth. Tell them they are settled and are part of the earth. Have them notice their soft and even breath. Tell them to imagine that they are growing from a seed. Have them imagine that from their heart, a beautiful flower is growing and opening up toward the warm sun above them. It is a vivid bright color, whatever their favorite color is. Its leaves are crisp and bright green, and its petals are so soft, they almost want to reach out and touch them. Tell them to feel warm beneath the sun, blowing in the breeze. After a few minutes, ring the chimes and ask the children to begin to wiggle their fingers and toes, then stretch and slowly roll over, and finally come up to a seated position.

Time: Five to Ten Minutes

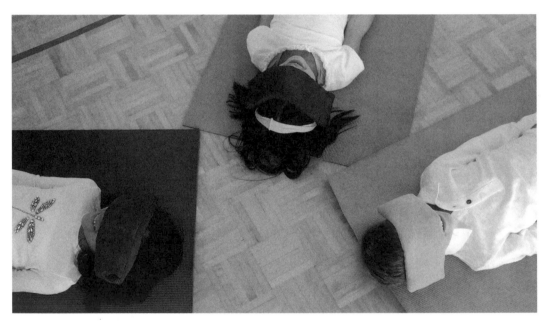

Figure 2.2. Meditation with herbal eye pillows

Gratitude: Invite the children to keep their eyes closed and place their hand on their knees, fingers in Earth mudra (ring finger pressed against thumb). This will make them feel patient and responsible. Ask them to silently be grateful for the abundant Earth and all the things that grow for them, giving them food, oxygen, and beauty. Ring the chimes and end by repeating, "Namaste, the light in me honors the light in you."

Time: Five to Ten Minutes

2.
Muscles

Seven- to Nine-Year-Olds

Educational Elements: Freedom of movement, language development, vocabulary enrichment, sensorial exploration to solidify concepts, promotion of grace and courtesy within the group

Props: Diagram of the human body that enables the children to see the various muscle groups, Popsicle sticks, small Styrofoam balls, colored modeling clay, one balloon, yoga mats, music, chimes

Intention: Invite the children to sit on their mats and welcome them to the class. Ringing the chimes gently will focus them. Tell them that for class they will discuss the muscles in their bodies. Discuss the fact that they have 640 muscles in their bodies. Show them a diagram of the muscles in a body, pointing out the biceps, deltoids, quadriceps, abdominals, dorsals, frontalis (forehead), and of course the gluteus maximus. Have them identify these muscles on their own bodies. Tell them that they are going to use these muscles today. Invite further discussion.

Time: Five to Ten Minutes

Warm-Up: Begin in a seated position and warm up the face muscles by having the kids smile, frown, look surprised, widen their mouths, and wiggle their ears. Invite them to make different faces, noticing the muscles they use. Then begin a flow of poses (see vinyasa 1, page 203).

Time: Approx. Five Minutes

Connect: Balloon bumping. Send one balloon around your circle of children several times. Each time the balloon goes around, ask the children to use one set of muscles only to pass the balloon along (e.g., they can only use their biceps for one round, then their abdominals, then their gluteus maximus). Encourage them to keep the balloon from touching the floor as it goes around.

Time: Five to Ten Minutes

Activity: Dance and move. Ask the children to scatter around the room. Turn on some fast-paced music and have the children dance and move freely. Turn off the music and ask them to go into a particular pose (e.g., warrior). While they hold the pose, ask them what muscles they feel they are working most in their bodies. Most will say

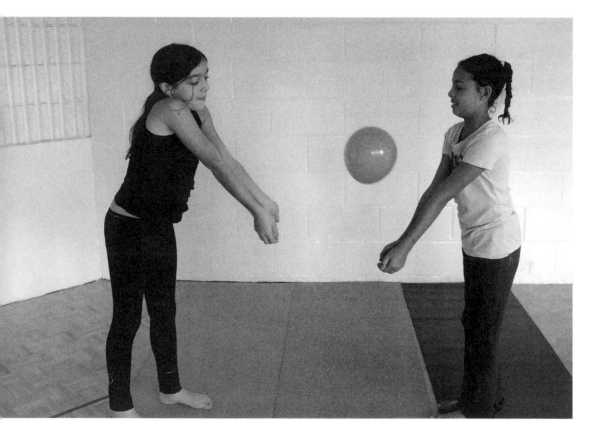

Figure 2.3. Balloon bumping

their quadriceps. Then turn the music back on and have them dance again. Stop the music and guide the children into another pose (e.g., boat pose). Notice if the children point out that their abdominals are working hard now. Continue on in this way, calling out different poses throughout the activity that isolate certain muscle groups.

Time: Ten to Fifteen Minutes

Arts and Crafts: The muscle man. Have one muscle man ready to go for each child. Use sticks (Popsicle sticks are good) for a body frame and attach a little Styrofoam ball to the top for a head. Give the children each a little ball of red modeling clay. Tell them to make one muscle group at a time from their modeling clay—for example, the quadriceps or the deltoids. They should mold the muscles and then place them on their muscle man until he is covered in muscles. Have a diagram of the muscles of the body handy for the kids' reference as you proceed.

Time: Ten to Fifteen Minutes

Meditation: Ring the chimes, gong, or whatever you are using today and have the children gather on their mats for their final relaxation. Invite them to lie on their backs, with their chins tilted slightly down toward their chests. Dim the lights and play light music. Talk the children through a body scan, having them flex and relax their toe muscles. Have them flex their heels and then relax them. Have them point their toes, feeling their quads as they do so, and then relax their legs, letting them sink into the mat like goo. Ask them to squeeze their gluteus maximus and then relax it, then flex and relax their abs. Proceed all the way up the body in this way to the facial muscles. Enjoy a few minutes of silence, and then ring the chimes to end the meditation. Invite the children to stretch, roll over, and return to a seated position.

Time: Approx. Ten Minutes

Creative Yoga for Children

Gratitude: Encourage the children to try the tall house mudra by pressing their middle fingers gently to their thumbs. Then have them close their eyes. Tell them that this mudra helps all the joints and the muscles in their bodies work well. Ask them to feel grateful for their strong bodies that let them move however they need to. Everyone can now repeat together, "Namaste, the light in me honors the light in you."

Time: Five to Ten Minutes

3.

Fun with Words

Seven- to Nine-Year-Olds

Educational Elements: Language development, freedom of movement, sensorial exploration in order to solidify abstract notions

Props: Twenty-six-page booklets of blank paper for each member of your group, larger pieces of paper (one for each child) for the acrostics activity, one ball of yarn, markers or colored pencils, stapler for the booklets, Tibetan singing bowl, yoga mats, music

Intention: Gather the children in a circle, and strike a Tibetan singing bowl or chimes to indicate the beginning of the class. With the children settled on their mats, tell them that for class, they will talk about words and all the fun they can have with them. Ask them what they can do with words—words can make stories or poems, games like hangman, or puzzles like word search. Elicit conversation from your group.

Time: Five to Ten Minutes

Warm-Up: Guide the children through a short flow of warm-up poses (see vinyasa 2, page 203).

Time: Five to Ten Minutes

Connect 1: Making a story. Make up a story using a pose in each sentence. For example, you may begin with the sentence, "One day a pigeon went for a walk." You can demonstrate the pigeon pose following the sentence. The next child can add to the story using a unique pose, for example, they may say, "The pigeon rested under a

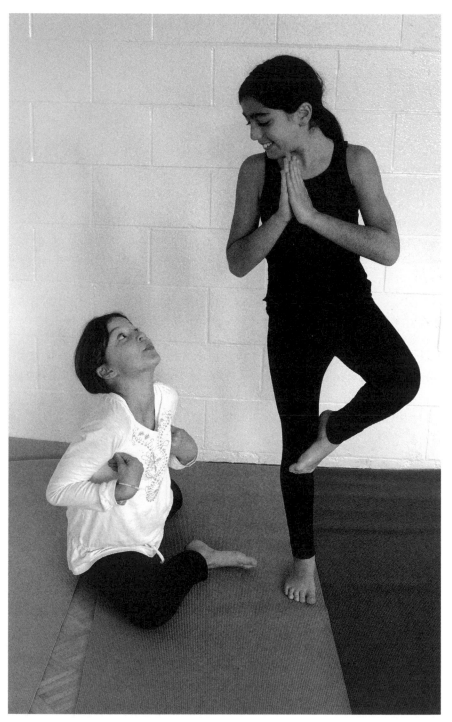

Figure 2.4. Making a story

tree." That child can then demonstrate the tree pose. Continue on in this way, having each child add to the story using a yoga pose as part of his or her idea until you have a complete story that you have made together as a group.

Time: Five to Ten Minutes

Connect 2: Web of names. Have a ball of yarn in your hand and explain that you are going to demonstrate a pose that begins with the first letter of your name (e.g., if your name is Adrienne, do the alligator pose). After you do the pose, hold on to one end of the yarn and toss it across the circle to a child. He can then do a pose, for example, if his name is David, he can do the downward dog pose. In turn, he should keep hold of one end of the yarn and toss it across to the next person. Continue on in this way until everyone has had a turn, and the web of wool has been created, crossing back and forth across the circle. You can then all stand up carefully, lifting the web you have created together, admiring it. You can release it if you like.

Time: Approx. Ten Minutes

Activity: Acrostics. Give each child a piece of paper and something to write with. Ask them to write their name vertically down their page.

Each child can write the name of a pose beginning with each letter of his or her name and later present it to the group, demonstrating the poses on the list as a little flow.

Time: Ten to Fifteen Minutes

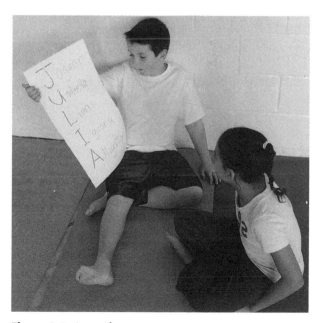

Figure 2.5. Acrostics

Arts and Crafts: Yoga dictionary. Distribute little booklets with twenty-six pages (prestapled or have the children staple the pages). Have the children create their own dictionary, drawing poses for each letter of the alphabet, one pose per page. Children can also take these books home and finish them at their own pace.

Time: Ten to Fifteen Minutes

Partner Pose: Taffy pull. Pair up the children and introduce them to the taffy pull pose (refer to partner pose 12, page 192).

Time: Approx. Five Minutes

Meditation: Ring the Tibetan singing bowl and gather their children for their final relaxation. Dim the lights and put soft music on. Ask them to close their eyes, lie on their backs, and have their hands fall down to their sides. Ask them to imagine that they are on magic carpets flying through the sky. Ask them to imagine that they see birds in the sky. Ask them to imagine what kind of birds they see—perhaps they are red or brown, or they are sleek or puffy, or they have sharp beaks or pointy claws. Ask them to then imagine how the birds are flying—perhaps they are flying quickly, slowly, powerfully, or angrily. Use lots of adjectives about your birds and lots of adverbs about how they move. Continue your visualization, perhaps talking about seeing stars, clouds, or planes on your journey, always including adjectives and adverbs for vivid descriptions. Finally, tell the children to bring their magic carpets in for a landing. Have them stretch, roll over, and come up to a seated position with their hands on their knees, cross-legged, palms facing up.

Time: Approx. Ten Minutes

Gratitude: Ask the children to be silently grateful for their wonderful minds and their great imaginations. Tell them that anything is possible as long as they can use their strong imaginations.

End the class by repeating, "Namaste, the light in me honors the light inside of you."

Time: Five to Ten Minutes

4.6
Zoology

Seven- to Nine-Year-Olds

Educational Elements: Freedom of choice, freedom of movement, sensorial exploration, language enrichment, grace, and courtesy and cooperation within the group

Props: Precut cardboard; blank puzzles pieces for each child in the class; markers or coloring pencils; individual paper cards with stick figure representations of the animal poses together with the associated animals on them that also indicate whether the animal a vertebrate, invertebrate, omnivore, herbivore, or carnivore; gong; music; yoga mats

Intention: Gather the children around and use a different device such as a gong in order to start the class. Perhaps give each of them a chance to strike the gong themselves. When the children are seated on their mats, explain the word "zoology" to them and how it is the study of animals. Explain what carnivores, herbivores, and finally omnivores are and see if the children can give you examples of animals from each group. Tell the children that today's activities will include animals from these groups.

Time: Five to Ten Minutes

Warm-Up: Using straps (belts or scarves can work) show the children how to wind the ends around their hands, leaving a horizontal, shoulder-width measure of strap between their hands. Have them stretch their arms out in front of them and, as they inhale, raise their straps above their heads, stretching their arms as high as they can.

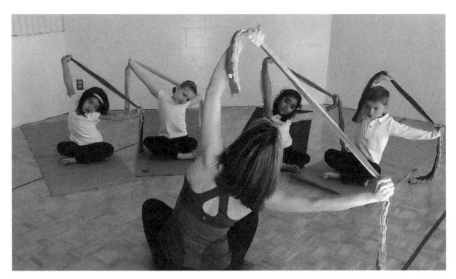

Figure 2.6. Warm-up with straps

As they exhale, have them bend their elbows so that the strap lowers behind their heads, squeezing their shoulder blades together. Have them feel their lungs get bigger and wider as they breathe. On the inhalation they can raise their arms up again toward the ceiling, and then as they exhale, they should lower them down in front of their chests onto their laps, all the while keeping their strap taught. Do this exercise for a few minutes, and then have the children put the straps aside and do a few sun salutations.

Time: Five to Ten Minutes

Connect: Marble massage. Hand out two marbles to each child and ask them to roll them around under each foot. Tell them to notice how the marbles feel under the balls of their feet, then the arches, and then their heels. Next, ask the children to work together to bring the marbles to the middle of the room. They must transport them by squeezing them between their toes, crab walking them to the middle of the circle, and dropping them into a communal bowl.

Time: Five to Ten Minutes

Activity: Animal dance. Have a collection of animal pose cards prepared for the children to choose out of a container. Some can be carnivores (e.g., lion, wolf, panther), some can be herbivores (e.g., rabbit, camel, elephant), and some can be omnivores (e.g., flamingo, raccoon, crow). Have the children notice whether their card also says V for vertebrate or I for invertebrate, and discuss what these words mean. Explain that they will all move around the room while the music is playing in the way that their animal would move (e.g., the cobra, being a vertebrate and a carnivore, would slide and slither). Play some fast-paced music, and when you turn it off, ask the children to freeze. Call out the name of one of the animals (e.g., frog). The child who has this animal can demonstrate their animal's movement, and everyone can try this. Ask the children to tell you if the animal is a vertebrate or invertebrate. They can also tell you what kind of vertebrate the frog is (e.g., amphibian) and whether the frog is a carnivore, omnivore, or herbivore. Turn the music back on and have the children move freely again. Continue on with game until everyone has had a turn. The children will come up with all sorts of information to share about the animals as they play the game.

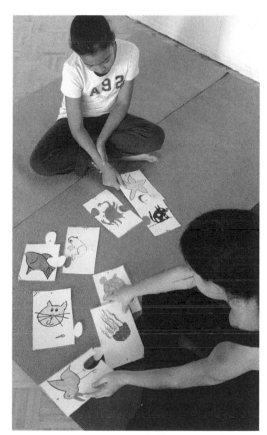

Figure 2.7. Invertebrate/vertebrate puzzles

Time: Approx. Fifteen Minutes

Arts and Crafts: Minipuzzles. Hand out blank cardboard minipuzzles (you can find these premade). You can make them yourself using Bristol board and dividing it into six to twelve pieces. Ask the children to draw an animal you have talked about in the class in each of the pieces of their blank puzzle. They can draw the animal (e.g., horse) and then label it with the letter V for vertebrate, O for omnivore, and H for herbivore. When completed, the children will have their own puzzle of animals. Display the cards used in the previous game for the children's reference when they are drawing their animals on their puzzles.

Time: Ten to Fifteen Minutes

Partner Pose: Double downward dog. Refer to partner pose 4, page 190.

Time: Five to Ten Minutes

Meditation: Strike your gong, chime, or singing bowl and ask the children to gather for their final meditation. Dim the lights and put on soft music. Ask them to lie on their backs with their chins tilted slightly down toward their chests. They can let their arms hang at their sides, with palms turned upward. Ask them to sink into their mats and to imagine that they are on a train ride through a wild forest. Point out all the animals that they see along their journey, and have them notice what these animals are eating and what they are doing. Try to include the animals you have discussed in class. At the end of the visualization, tell the children that the train is pulling into the station, and the ride is coming to an end. It is now the end of the day and the sun is going down. Pause for a minute or two, and then ask the children to begin to wiggle their fingers and toes, then stretch, and finally roll over and come into a seated position with their hands to their hearts. Ask them to feel their breath going in and out of their nose. Gently strike the gong.

Time: Five to Ten Minutes

Gratitude: Ask the children to be silently thankful for our beautiful world, full of so many forms of animals. Each animal relies on other species to coexist in order to keep the food chain going and to survive. Humanity is part of that coexistence, and we should value that.

End the class with "Namaste, the light inside of me honors the light inside of you."

Time: Five to Ten Minutes

5.

The Body Systems

Seven- to Nine-Year-Olds

Educational Elements: Language enrichment, grace, courtesy and cooperation, sensorial exploration and movement used to solidify abstract educational concepts

Props: One rope fifteen feet in length and another five feet in length, cut-outs in the shape of a human body (enough for each child), large sheet of paper for you to draw a body on, markers or colored pencils, music, herbal eye pillows, chimes, yoga mats, premade names of body parts and their definitions (enough for one for each child)

Intention: Gather the children in a circle on their mats and ring the chimes to begin the class. Tell them that for class, they are going to think about how all the parts of their bodies are interconnected. Just how people all have to work together to get things accomplished, so does the body. When they eat a piece of food, that food has to travel through many parts of the body that break it down. This is called the digestive system. The children will have some ideas for you on how that system works. Have a discussion, mentioning that everyone has a nervous system, a circulatory system, and so on.

Time: Five to Ten Minutes

Warm-Up: Tell the children that they will start the warm-up by stretching their eyes first. Ask them to sit cross-legged and hold their arm out in front of them, thumb raised to the sky and level with their chin. Ask them to imagine that they are resting their chin on the edge of a table

Creative Yoga for Children

and they cannot move it. Now they should move their arm in a huge circle in front of them, following the thumb with their eyes without moving their heads at all. See if they can do it clockwise a few times and then counterclockwise a few times. When their eyes feel warmed up, they can come into table position (hands and knees on the mat, shoulder distance apart). Instruct the class that they will now begin a vinyasa (see vinyasa 2, page 203).

Time: Five to Ten Minutes

Connect: Intestine walking! Gather the children and stretch out a cord along the floor that is approximately fifteen feet in length. Tell them that this represents how long their small intestines are. Stretch out another cord that is five feet in length on the floor, pointing out that this is about the length of their large intestines, which are a lot thicker than their small intestines but are actually much shorter. Have the children connect the two cords as they are connected in the body.

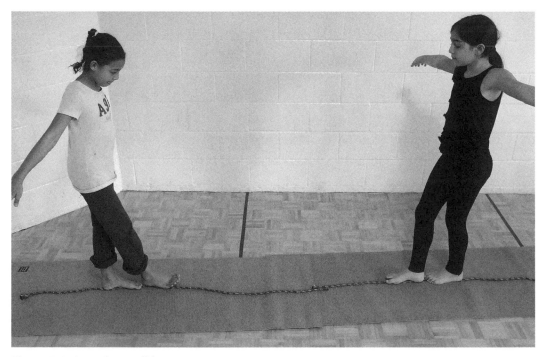

Figure 2.8. Intestine walking

Have them walk on the rope, one at a time, for its entire length. They will be excited to learn that this is the same distance that it would take to walk across their own intestines!

Time: Five to Ten Minutes

Activity: What's my function? Before the class begins, compose a list of internal organs (e.g., stomach, intestines, bladder, kidneys, liver, heart, lungs) and a write them down on individual cards. Then compose a list of definitions for those parts (e.g., for the heart, write, "Pumps blood through the body," or for lungs write, "Fills the blood with oxygen as it pumps through") and write these on another set of cards. Make the definitions fairly basic. Hand out the "body parts" to half of your class and the definitions to the other half (or have them draw from a hat). The children can read them out and you can assist them in finding their matching person. As you read through the definitions and parts, draw them on a large sheet of paper so the children actually see where their body part exists in their bodies. Encourage lots of group discussion with this activity.

Time: Approx. Fifteen Minutes

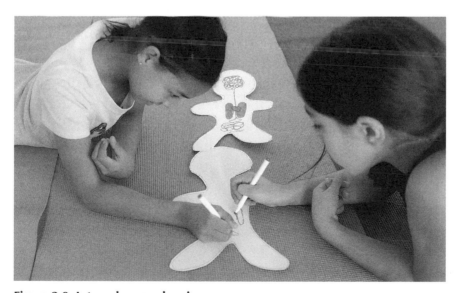

Figure 2.9. Internal organ drawings

Breath: Hoberman breathing. Take some time now for the children to relax and pass a Hoberman sphere around the circle. As they inhale, they can open up the sphere all the way with their hands and feel their lungs and belly open up, too. As they exhale, they will close the sphere and feel everything in their body empty out and actually get smaller. Each child should take a few breaths and pass the sphere around.

Time: Approx. Five Minutes

Arts and Crafts: The amazing body. Review the body parts and their functions with the children, showing them your illustration of this. Give each child a sheet of paper that has been cut out to look like a human body outline. The children can then draw and color in the organs within the body, referring to your drawing for help. They can add their own colorful touches, like drawing food in the stomach, blood pumping through the heart, and so on.

Time: Ten to Fifteen Minutes

Partner Pose: Twist and turn. The children can now practice the twist and turn pose (refer to partner pose 8, page 191). They can practice this with the child that they matched up with in the previous activity.

Time: Approx. Five Minutes

Meditation: Ring your chimes and have the children relax on their mats for a final meditation. Dim the lights and put on soft music. Perhaps give out herbal eye pillows if they would like. Begin telling a story, asking the children to imagine that they are travelling through the body. Ask them to imagine that they are a piece of their favorite food. They enter the mouth, are swallowed, and travel down to the stomach. They see other parts of the body on their way. They see blood that is blue (nonoxygenated), and blood that is red (oxygenated) carried around through long veins. They see organs (liver, kidneys, pancreas), muscles, and bones. Add your own elements to this story. Finally, have a few minutes of silence; ring the chimes; and have the children stretch, roll over, and come back up to a seated position. They can place their hands in the water mudra, with their baby finger pressed against their thumbs. Tell them that this mudra keeps all the liquid and water in their bodies flowing freely.

Time: Approx. Ten Minutes

Gratitude: Ask the children to be silently grateful for their health. Ask them to be grateful for the miracle that is their body. Ask them to wonder at how all its parts seem to know how to work together and how to connect, relying on one another and helping each other as people do in their lives. End by repeating, "Namaste, the light within me honors the light within you."

Time: Five to Ten Minutes

6.

Countries of the World

Seven- to Nine-Year-Olds

Educational Elements: Grace and courtesy, cooperation, freedom of movement, sensorial exploration, language enrichment, refinement of movement, balance and coordination

Props: Two Bristol boards (one for drawing a control map of the continents and oceans and the second for drawing the same but cut it out into separate pieces), hoops, stamp pads, stampers that illustrate poses or stickers with poses drawn on them, music, a globe, chimes, small blank passport booklets cut out of construction paper, atlas

Intention: Gather the children by using your gong, chimes, or singing bowl. Talk to the children about the globe. Have one available to pass around. Talk about what separates the countries and continents from one another (e.g., oceans, land borders). Ask the children how many countries they think are in the world. Point out the continents. Tell them that they will be exploring the world today. Encourage the children's input (e.g., have them show each other some of the countries they have been to and how they got there).

Time: Five to Ten Minutes

Warm-Up: Start in table position, going into cat stretch, and then cow. Then begin a vinyasa (see vinyasa 3, page 203).

Time: Five to Ten Minutes

Connect: Where in the world. Give each child a picture of either a continent or an ocean of the world (cut these out from construction paper beforehand). Display a large drawing of a map of the world (just outlines of continents and oceans) on the floor in front of the children. Ask the children to one at a time look at the map on the floor and then place their piece of the world where it goes (superimposing it). Each child places his or her puzzle piece where it goes, and then they name it together. Finally, the world is complete and you have made it together!

Time: Approx. Ten Minutes

Activity: Passport game. In advance of the class, make each child a little blank passport made of construction paper (a stapled paper booklet with eight blank pages). Tell them that they are travelling and they need to stamp their passport as they arrive at each stop they are visiting. Place eight hula hoops around your room, with a stamp or a sticker in each showing a pose (e.g., dog or cat pose). Place an ink pad in the hoop as well if you are using stampers. The children will travel (dance) around the room as you play music, and when you turn it off, they should stop in a hula hoop and do the pose that they find there. When they have done the pose, they can stamp their passport or place the sticker of the pose in the passport. They are then ready to travel again and stop at a new hula hoop. As the music plays, you may suggest that the children change the way they travel. They can pretend to fly, travel in a boat, or move as a land creature. Continue on in this way until the children have visited all the hula hoops and have filled their passports.

Time: Approx. Fifteen Minutes

Breath: Ring your chimes and have the children come back to their mats. Tell them they must be tired after their journey around the world, so you are all going to make lemonade. Have them stretch their legs out and pretend to squeeze imaginary lemons with their toes to make their drinks. They can then draw their feet up toward their mouths, pretending to hold their lemonade. Ask them to stick out their tongues and shape them into a straw, then pretend to sip the lemonade as they inhale, and just exhale normally. This straw-sipping breath will cool them down. Practice it five or six times.

Time: Five Minutes

Book: *Children's Atlas of the World* by Chez Picthall and Christiane Gunzi. As the children find a place on the globe, they can then point it out in the atlas.

Time: Five to Ten Minutes

Meditation: Dim the lights now and play very soft music. The children can come into corpse pose. In corpse pose, children are lying down on their backs with their eyes closed, arms down by their sides and palms facing upwards. Tell them to just let their feet flop out.

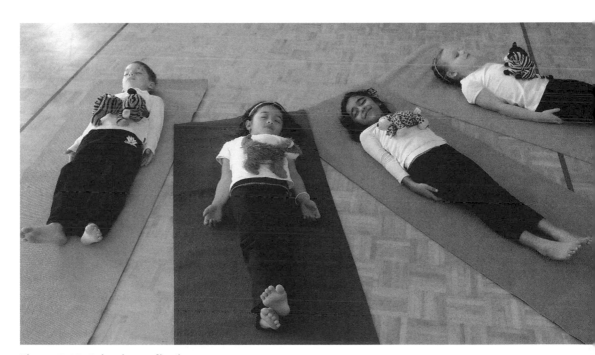

Figure 2.10. Lying in meditation

Place a stuffed animal on each child's belly and ask the children to keep very still, as they are going to take this "friend" on a flight across the earth, and if they are not still, this friend will fall off. Tell the children to sink into their mats and to take off on their flight around the world. Tell them they are floating and ask them to imagine that they see an ocean below them. Perhaps there are ships, jumping dolphins, or spouting whales below. Tell them they are crossing over North America next, pointing out mountains, rivers, and deserts. Continue having them travel the earth over different continents. Finally, tell the children that they have crossed the earth, and they are landing now. Have them stretch slowly, roll over, and come up into a seated position, hands in a prayer position and eyes closed.

Time: Five to Ten Minutes

Gratitude: Ask the children now to be silently grateful for their ability to practice yoga together with their friends and to silently send positive energy and love to all the other children in the places around the world that they have visited today.

End with "Namaste, the light in me honors the light in you."

Time: Five to Ten Minutes

7.

The Creation
of the Universe

Seven- to Nine-Year-Olds

Educational Elements: Learning abstract concepts through the senses, freedom of movement, freedom of expression and choice, language enrichment, cooperation and grace, and courtesy

Props: Large drawing of the solar system for the children's reference as they create their craft, several pipe cleaners, various-sized Styrofoam balls (enough to give ten to each child), markers, music, yoga mats, chimes, herbal eye pillows

Intention: Gather the children using chimes, a singing bowl, or a gong. When they are seated on their mats, tell them that they will talk about the big bang that happened about fourteen billion years ago. Explain that the big bang was a big explosion that created the matter that created the whole universe. Discuss what the children know about this. From the big bang came the matter that created planets, meteors, stars, and galaxies. All the force that came from that big bang is still moving around, and as a result, the universe is expanding.

Time: Five to Ten Minutes

Warm-Up: We are all matter. Have the children form a tight little ball on their mats—tell them they are a piece of matter in space. Ask them to inhale, and then on the exhalation, they can get bigger until they explode into the air, stretching their hands and feet apart.

In a standing position, begin to do a few sun salutations and then a vinyasa (see vinyasa 5, page 203).

Time: Five Minutes

Connect: The big bang. Come together hand in hand in a circle. Tell the children that they are all gas coming together, but the big bang is coming soon. With you leading, let go of one child's hand and lead the children into a tight spiral circle, everyone walking together, the circle getting tighter. Then say, "Bang!" Have everyone come apart and roll away from the middle. Tell the children they can pick what they want to become: a star, a planet, a meteor, a galaxy, a nebula, a black hole, a quasar, and so on. They can call it out and take their place somewhere in the room. Observe the children now and tell them that they have created the universe. Have them each identify to the class what they have become. Have the children remain in their places; this activity leads directly into the next one.

Time: Five to Ten Minutes

Activity: The gravity dance. Assign each child a role as a planet, moon, or asteroid. Gradually, gravity will pull them all together to form solar systems. You as the teacher are "gravity," and you will pull everyone together into their place. Wander around the room, and as you tap each child, he or she will follow you to a new place to stand. The "sun" will be in the middle of the room and everyone will take their positions in relation to the sun. When everyone is in their place, turn on some music and have everyone orbit around the sun. The moons will orbit around their planets. Asteroids can move more freely in and out. Everyone must "rotate" as they move as well as orbit. This is the gravity dance. Have a big picture drawn beforehand of the solar system, and display it for the children's reference.

Time: Ten to Fifteen Minutes

Arts and Crafts: Solar system swirls. The children will create their own solar system using long pipe cleaners (two pipe cleaners connected together for each child is ideal). They will all receive nine varied sizes of Styrofoam balls, plus one larger one that will be the sun. Ask them to color these balls in the colors they would like to form all the planets. When finished, they can begin to pierce the end of their pipe cleaner through the sun first, as if they are sewing and the pipe cleaner is their needle and thread. After the sun, ask them to slide Mercury onto their pipe cleaner and slide it along, leaving a space between it and the sun. Then they can add Venus, then Earth, and gradually all the planets will be attached to the pipe cleaner. They can then begin to coil the pipe cleaner around and around, with the sun in the exact middle. When finished, they will have created their own solar system swirl. Use a picture of the solar system that shows the planets on the axis in order to guide the children.

Time: Ten to Fifteen Minutes

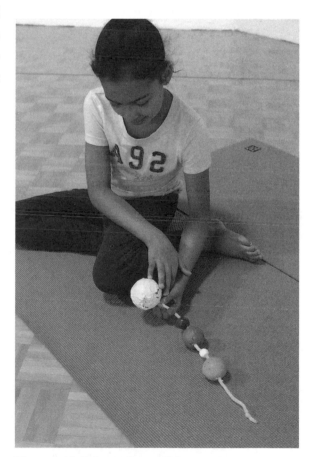

Figure 2.11. Solar system swirls

Meditation: Ring your chimes/gong. Ask the children to relax on their mats, lying down for their final relaxation time. Ask them to close their eyes, tilt their chins slightly in toward their chests, let their palms open up to the sky, and have their feet flop out to the sides. Dim the lights and put on relaxing music. They may use herbal eye pillows if they would like. Tell the children that they are in their own private rocket ship, cozy and warm, and there is no gravity on the ship, so they feel weightless. They have a little porthole window to gaze out of as they travel away from Earth. The sky outside is black, and the stars twinkle brightly, one at a time. Point out various planets that they are passing. Point out moons, volcanoes, and craters that they see on them. The objects they pass are so bright, they feel like they can almost reach out and touch them. Ask the children to notice if they can hear any sounds in space. Continue on, adding to your story of their rocket ship journey. Finally, have them return to Earth, coming in for a landing on the ocean. Their spacecraft floats up and down in the ocean, drifting to the shore. Enjoy a few silent minutes at the end, then ring the chimes. Ask the children to stretch, roll over to one side, and come to a seated position on their mats.

Time: Five to Ten Minutes

Gratitude: Ask the children to sit now with their eyes closed and silently give thanks for their perfect planet. It is not too hot or too cold and it is just the right distance away from the sun. It is full of oxygen for them to breathe and has the perfect weather, unlike all the other planets. Tell them they should be thankful for this and must preserve their Earth. End with "Namaste, the light in me honors the light inside of you."

Time: Five to Ten Minutes

8.

Drama/Performance

Seven- to Nine-Year-Olds

Educational Elements: Development of self-confidence through movement, cooperation, sensorial exploration, and the freedom of choice; language enrichment; grace and courtesy

Props: A gong, chimes, or a singing bowl; a mandala that you either bring in or make yourself; large sheets of drawing paper (one sheet per child); markers or colored pencils; book (*Ish* by Peter Reynolds); stuffed animals (one for each child); yoga mats; music; pose cards and partner pose cards and a bag to keep them in

Intention: Gather the children on their mats by using the chimes. Ask them if they enjoy acting and performing in plays. Talk about different ways of performing, whether it be through public speaking, acting, or dancing. Tell them there are many ways of publically expressing themselves and ask them to name a few examples. Tell them that they will do some performing as well as practicing various methods that let them perform better.

Time: Five to Ten Minutes

Warm-Up: Have the children sit cross-legged on their mats in a comfortable way (half lotus, perhaps). Tell them they are going to warm up their faces, voices, and ears. Have the kids open up their mouths as wide as they can, stick out their tongues, move it around, and make "Aaa" noises. Have the kids make different expressions (e.g., happiness, sadness, shock, anger, or sleepiness). Have them wiggle their ears, do some neck rolls, and blink their eyes. Then do a little vinyasa of poses to warm up the rest of the body.

Time: Five to Ten Minutes

Connect: Mirroring. Have the children divide into groups of two or three. Ask one person to move his hands slowly up and down in front of him, and the other child(ren) will copy him exactly, as if looking into a mirror. Have them explore moving their face, arms, legs, and so on. Then switch and let the next child be the leader of the actions.

Time: Five to Ten Minutes

Activity: Pose plays. Divide the children up into groups of three or four, depending on your class size. Offer the children to choose one pose card each from a bag. They can also choose as a group one or two partner pose cards. Have the children go off into their groups privately for a few minutes to plan a little play. They will act as the characters they have chosen (e.g., cat, mermaid, or alligator). They must use all their poses in their play. After some planning time, the groups will return and present their plays to the class. There will be much laughter and silliness during this fun activity.

Time: Approx. Fifteen Minutes

Arts and Crafts: Mandala making. Tell the children that they are going to make mandalas in class. These are beautiful drawings that ancient yogis used to help them focus as they meditated. These are still used by people today and are great tools to use to help everyone focus and relax before a play, a performance, a speech, and so on. Have a mandala predrawn and show it to the children. There should be a small focal point drawn right in the center of the design (e.g., an eye or a star) and then shapes drawn around it that encircle it, getting bigger and bigger, until the page is entirely designed. The point of the mandala is to draw the eye right in the center. Let the children freely design their own mandalas that they can use whenever they like.

Time: Ten to Fifteen Minutes

Book: *Ish* by Peter Reynolds. This is a wonderful and inspiring book about the beauty and value of one's own uniqueness and one's own self-expression. You can read this during or after the mandala-making exercise.

Time: Five Minutes

Partner Pose: Partner tree. After the plays, pair the children off to try this partner pose (refer to partner pose 9, page 191).

Time: Five to Ten Minutes

Meditation: Ring the chimes, gong, or singing bowl and gather the children for their final relaxation. They can lie down on their backs and close their eyes. Place a little stuffed animal on each child's

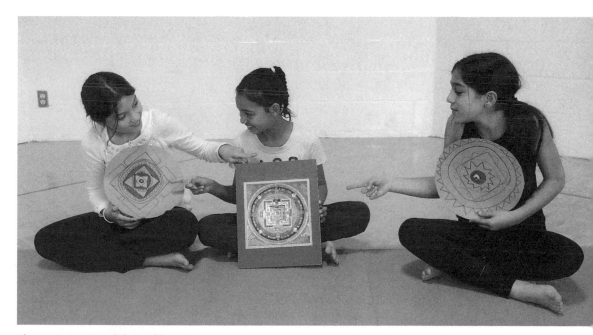

Figure 2.12. Mandala making

stomach, and tell the children that this little companion is going to support them as they do a grand performance for the world. The stuffed animals must rise up and down with the children's breath, because breathing deeply is so important when they are performing. Tell them they are on a grand stage with big lights trained on them. There are thousands of people in the audience. They are giving their greatest performance ever, but they feel confident and secure. Tell them they are focused and relaxed. Have the children imagine what their performance is (dancing, acting, singing, etc.) Their little friend is right there with them, making sure they are breathing calmly. Talk through this little visualization and tell the children to feel proud of themselves when it is over. Tell them they can accomplish anything. After a few silent minutes, ring the chimes and have the children stretch and move. They can come up to a seated position gradually, keeping their eyes closed.

Time: Five to Ten Minutes

Gratitude: Ask the children to silently give thanks for the support their friends and family give them in their lives. Ask them to feel grateful that they have the tools and the ability to do anything they want to do in their lives. End with "Namaste, the light in me honors the light inside of you."

Time: Five to Ten Minutes

9.

Shapes and Angles

Seven- to Nine-Year-Olds

Educational Elements: Development of self-confidence through movement, cooperation, sensorial exploration, and the freedom of choice; language of mathematics; geometry; grace and courtesy

Props: Several tooth picks and Popsicle sticks, construction paper (enough for one sheet per child), glue, large picture of all the shapes that they will make for the class, yoga mats, music, chimes, herbal eye pillows (optional)

Intention: Gather the children using the chimes and have them sit comfortably on their mats. Welcome them to yoga. Explain that they will be talking about shapes that they see in the world—some have a few sides and some have many sides. For example, ask them how many sides the following shapes have: triangle, square, pentagon, hexagon, and so on. Ask them if there are objects that they see every day that have these shapes (e.g., a piece of pizza is a triangle, a book is usually a rectangle, a stop sign is an octagon). The children will have many ideas. Draw these multisided shapes on a large sheet of paper for the children to see as you discuss them. Tell them that all these multisided shapes are called polygons.

Time: Five to Ten Minutes

Warm-Up: Begin by curling up in a little ball on the mat, telling the children that you are a circle, but you are going to change shape because you are a shape-shifter. Stand up and turn yourself into a straight line, then open your legs and become a triangle. Ask the children to turn themselves into squares now—they will all have different ways of doing this. Do a few more shapes, and then begin a little warm-up flow of postures.

Time: Five to Ten Minutes

Connect: Sticking together. Gather the children into a circle and have ten Popsicle sticks in a pile in front of you. Tell the children that they are going to work together, using only their feet, to pass these sticks, one by one, around the circle. Send the first stick around the circle. Have the children be seated with legs stretched out in front to hold the stick as it comes to them. When the stick reaches the last child, he or she can lay it flat in the middle of the circle for all to see. As each stick comes to that child, he or she can connect it to the last stick in the center. At the end of the activity, the sticks will form a ten-sided figure, or a "decagon."

Time: Five to Ten Minutes

Activity: Human polygons. Tell the children that they are going to make shapes and angles using their bodies. Invite one child to make a line with his or her body. Invite another child create a right angle (lying on floor). Invite another child create an equilateral triangle (discuss what this is). Now have one child form an isosceles triangle and another form a scalene triangle. Some of the older children in the circle can explain to the younger ones what these are. Then use four children to make a square, then five for a pentagon, six for a hexagon, and so on. After everyone has had a turn, discuss the shapes they have made.

Time: Ten to Fifteen Minutes

Breath: Do a cooling alternate nostril breathing exercise with the children after this busy activity (see breathing exercise 3, page 205).

Time: Five Minutes

Arts and Crafts: Stick shapes. Have several toothpicks (or Popsicle sticks), construction paper, and glue on hand. The children can create their own displays of the shapes they made today using the sticks provided. They can simply stick them onto the paper and label each shape.

Time: Ten to Fifteen Minutes

Partner Pose: The Box. Divide the children up into pairs now and practice the box pose (see partner pose 11, page 192).

Time: Five Minutes

Meditation: Ring the chimes. Invite the children to relax on their mats for their final relaxation. Dim the lights and put on very soft music. Ask the children to close their eyes with their palms facing up, fingers uncurled, and feet flopped out to the sides. Ask them to imagine that they have no shape to them at all and that they are just blobs, seeping out onto the mat in every direction like melting butter or syrup on a pancake. Now they can imagine that their blob bodies are being poured into a triangle-shaped cookie cutter and that they are forming this shape. They are now being poured into a square cookie cutter and so have taken its shape. Have them go through numerous shapes—pentagon, hexagon, and so on—until finally they are poured back onto their mats and have no more shape to them at all. They are completely relaxed. After a few minutes, ask the children to begin to stretch, wiggle, and move, then come up to a seated position on their mats with their eyes closed.

Time: Five to Ten Minutes

Gratitude: Ask the children to silently be thankful for this beautiful day and to be thankful to everyone else in the room for practicing yoga together. They should all feel lucky that they can work so well together to create the things that they like. End with "Namaste, the light inside of me honors the light inside of you."

Time: Five to Ten Minutes

10.
Animal, Vegetable, or Mineral

Seven- to Nine-Year-Olds

Educational Elements: Freedom of movement, freedom of expression, sensorial exploration used to solidify abstract concepts, language enrichment, grace and courtesy, cooperation

Props: A blob of goo or slime (you can find this at any dollar store), a spine made out of spools, yellow sticky notes, illustrated pose cards (for reference if needed), music, yoga mats, herbal eye pillows

Intention: Gather the children and welcome them to yoga. When they are settled, tell them that today they are going to talk about the three main things that they find here in the world. They are animals, vegetables, and minerals. Ask them to name some animals. Show them a little blob of goo and tell them, "Creatures with no spine or exoskeleton look something like this; these are invertebrates." Then show them an example of a spine (to create a spine, see class 14, The Skeleton in chapter 1). Tell them that animals with a spine are called vertebrates. They can name some. Then discuss another form of life called "vegetables." Talk about plants, flowers, and so on. Finally, discuss the other thing on Earth that is not alive: minerals. Discuss some minerals (e.g., rocks, buildings, or bicycles). The children will give you more examples.

Time: Five to Ten Minutes

Warm-Up: Instruct the children to lie on their backs on their mats with their hands across their chests. Ask them now to imagine they are an otter floating down a calm river. Ask the children to visualize the shoreline, trees, and forest creatures pass as they continue their journey. Now as they slowly float toward the shore, have them roll over and come into table position. Now begin a vinyasa (see vinyasa 6, page 204).

Time: Five to Ten Minutes

Connect: Circle of oms. Have everyone seated in a circle, holding hands. Tell them to close their eyes and repeat the word "om," which is the sacred sound of the universe and sounds like a vibration. Have them repeat it three times together and then be silent for a moment. Ask the children to see if they can feel the vibration of energy in the room while they are chanting. Have them breathe in deeply, then on the exhalation, say "om." Do this three times. Allow them to do this at their own pace. Let the sound be lengthy. The children will tell you that they felt the connecting vibration as well as heard the sound. They will find this very cool.

Time: Five Minutes

Activity 1: "Who am I?" game. Write out a series of labels on sticky notes. They will include animals (fish, cat, flamingo, etc.), vegetables (tree, Venus flytrap, lotus, etc.), and minerals (boat, crescent moon, gateway, etc.), all of which are poses. Put a sticky on each child's back. Choose a child and have the others demonstrate the pose for that child. Watching others demonstrate the pose, the child must then guess what pose they are. Repeat this for each child. Everyone has a turn guessing what they are, and be sure that they notice whether they are a vegetable, animal, or mineral.

Time: Ten to Fifteen Minutes

Activity 2: Freeze dance. The children can now scatter out across the room. Put on some fun dancing music. Let the children move and dance. Stop the music occasionally. Then using the labels assigned to each child in activity 1, you can call out "mineral," "vegetable," or "animal." Only those who have those labels will do their pose. You can add to this by making it more specific (e.g., all those animals who are vertebrates can do a pose)

Time: Approx. Ten Minutes

Breath: Gather the children for a relaxing breath now. The children will be very warm after their game, so have them sit and do a relaxing breathing exercise by curling their tongues in the shape of straws and inhaling through them. Then they can close their mouths and exhale through their noses. Do this several times.

Time: Five Minutes

Book: If time allows, read *My Quiet Place* by Douglas Wood.

Time: Five to Ten Minutes

Meditation: Ring the chimes to signal that you are now going to do a final relaxation. The children can close their eyes, lie down, and stretch out on their backs. Dim the lights and play very soft music. Ask the children to feel their shoulders broaden out onto the mat and feel the backs of their heads grow heavy. Tell them to breathe softly and to let everything that is heavy inside them slide off to the sides and roll off the mat. Tell them to feel like an invertebrate that has no shell or skeleton. They are gooey like the goo they looked at in class. Perhaps they are amoebas or a bacteria. Maybe they are a squids. Ask them to feel like they are floating with no shape—their shape is always changing. Tell them to imagine how it feels. Continue on with your visualization and then have the children be silent for a few minutes. Ring the chimes and have them begin to wiggle toes and fingers, stretch, and move. Maybe have them bring their knees into their chests, wrap their arms around themselves, and roll from side to side. Then have them come up to a seated position with their hands in their favorite mudra.

Time: Five to Ten Minutes

Gratitude: Ask the children to silently think about the different creatures and elements that they see around them in the world. They are all different and unique. Ask them to be thankful for the differences between everything, the uniqueness of it. Being all the same is not beneficial to them; they need to be different. All their differences combine to meet everyone's needs.

End with "Namaste, the light in me honors the light in you."

Time: Five to Ten Minutes

Part III:
Class Themes
Ten- to Twelve-Year-Olds

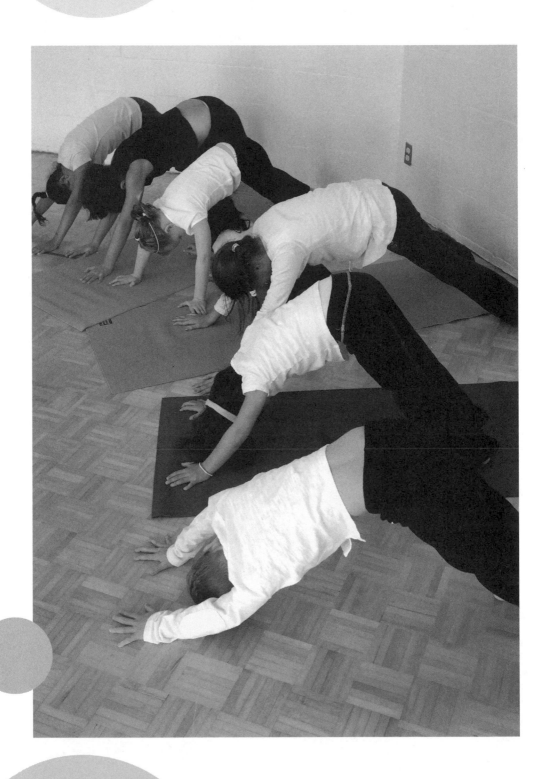

1.

Trust

Ten- to Twelve-Year-Olds

Educational Elements: Children exercising their own will and creativity, language enrichment, care of the person and development of self-respect, freedom of movement, learning through sensorial exploration

Props: Small ropes for each child in the class, enough bean bags for each pair of children to have twelve, blindfolds for half the number of children in the class, yoga mats, music, stuffed animals, chimes

Intention: Gather your group of children, signaling the start of the class with chimes, a gong, or a singing bowl. Begin a discussion about trust. Ask the children the following questions: Who are the people that we trust in our lives? When do we know we can trust someone? How do you earn someone's trust? Indicate to the children that today we will be doing activities that involve having to trust each other.

Time: Five to Ten Minutes

Warm-Up: Have the children stand in a circle and tell them they need to support one another to do a tree balance. They can go into a tree pose as a group, holding on to each other's shoulders. After this, lead them through a warm-up vinyasa of poses.

Time: Five to Ten Minutes

Connect: Create the shape. Give each child a length of string. The first child lays his or her string on the ground in the center of the circle. The shape is just a line. Tell them, "Let's see where we can go from here." The second person adds his or her string onto one end of the first person's, creating some sort of angle, which you can name. The third person has a turn, creating a triangle or a new side to the shape. Let the children build whatever they want and have them name their shape when they are finished.

Time: Approx. Ten Minutes

Activity 1: Building blind. Divide the children into groups of two to construct a pyramid that they will make out of bean bags. One of the children will provide instructions and the other will be the builder who will wear a blindfold. The children should start on one end of the

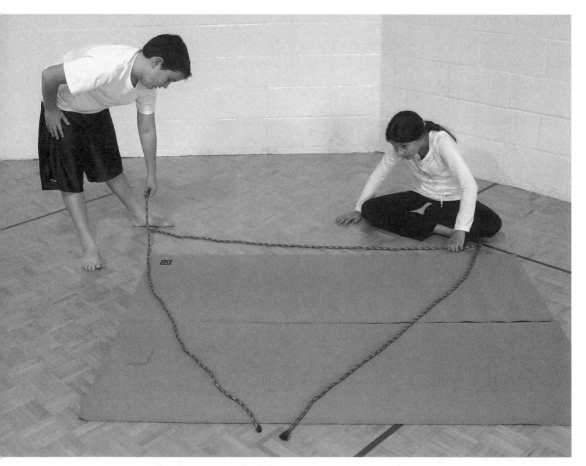

Figure 3.1. Creating the shape

room, blindfolded, and with the help of their partners, move across the room in a certain way (crab walking, penguin walking, etc.) in order to reach their bean bags. They will take a few bean bags and bring them back to their starting point and then must go back to get the rest. After they have collected all their bean bags, they can then begin building. The child giving the instructions will talk the builder through the construction of the pyramid without touching it at all. When the pyramids are built, the blindfolds can come off. Everyone can admire each other's pyramids, and then the partners can switch and the process can begin again.

Time: Approx. Fifteen Minutes

Activity 2: Willow in the wind. Ask the children to stand together in a close circle, with one child in the middle, blindfolded. Tell the children in the circle that they are going to be the wind and the child in the middle will be the willow tree, blowing through this wind. Have everyone outstretch their arms to touch the willow tree, who must be very trusting and lean on the others. The children gently pass the child

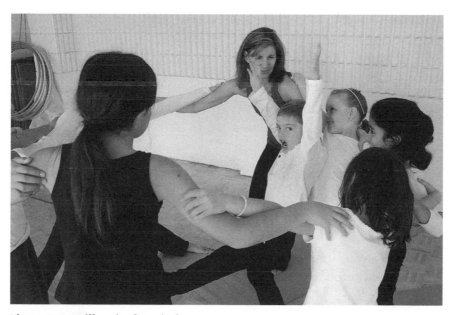

Figure 3.2. Willow in the wind

around the circle. As the willow tree child feels safer, he or she will be more trusting lean further and further into the group, creating a more fun ride! Give everyone who wants a turn a chance to be the willow tree.

Time: Ten Minutes

Partner Pose: The box. This pose involves a lot of trust (see partner pose 11, page 192).

Time: Five Minutes

Meditation: Ring the chimes and have the children return to their mats, lying down and closing their eyes for their final relaxation. Put on soft music and place stuffed beanie babies on the children's foreheads or bellies. Begin by asking the children to visualize that their stuffed toy trusts them not to let it fall to the ground. Tell them to imagine that they are lying on a tightrope, high up in the air over a forest, and they are perfectly balanced on this rope, as it runs underneath them, along their spine. Their bodies are exactly in the middle. Ask them to relax their shoulders, letting them sink, and spread their arms out with palms facing the sky. They can settle fully into the tightrope; their heads feel heavy. Even though the wind may blow around them, they can trust in the strength of this tightrope; they can trust that it will keep them safe and secure. But they must keep their little friend secure as well as balanced on them. Continue with this visualization for a minute or two, and then let the children have a few minutes of silence. Ring the chimes and have them roll over, stretch, and come into a seated position.

Time: Five to Ten Minutes

Gratitude: Ask the children to close their eyes with their hands to their hearts. Ask them to be silently grateful for those who they trust in their lives. Tell them that having someone's trust is a great gift but also a great responsibility and should be cherished. End with "Namaste, the light in me honors the light inside of you."

Time: Five to Ten Minutes

2.
Environmental Action

Ten- to Twelve-Year-Olds

Educational Elements: Freedom of movement, sensorial exploration, language enrichment, exercising of the child's will and imagination, environmental issues

Props: Canvas shopping bags (one for each child), pose cards or pose objects to put in each hoop, clues written out (one for each child) on ways to improve the environment, yoga mats, music, chimes, long string (two or three feet long), and two Styrofoam cups

Intention: Ring the chimes to gather your group together and have the children sit on their mats. Explain to them that today the class will discuss how they can feel empowered to make a difference in the world by preserving the environment. Discuss a few issues that are facing the environment today, like global warming, the ozone layer, and pollution.

Time: Five to Ten Minutes

Warm-Up: Begin with simple stretch in child's pose. Then begin a vinyasa (refer to vinyasa 2, page 203).

Time: Five to Ten Minutes

Connect: Sound waves. Tell the children that with this exercise, they can learn to work together as a group. This will help empower them to make real change in the world. Put together a long string that is connected to two cups, one on either end, like a makeshift telephone.

One child in the circle speaks into the cup, instructing the next child to do a certain pose (e.g., downward dog). The child on the receiving end of the phone may or may not hear it correctly but must do whatever pose he or she receives. Then the child who has given the instruction tosses the cup to a new child in the circle, and the child who just received the instruction then gives of the instruction to the new child. Continue on in this way until each child has given an instruction and has performed a pose. Afterward, talk about how this listening exercise went.

Time: Approx. Ten Minutes

Activity: Save the earth. Hand out a small canvas shopping bag (you can get these at the dollar store) to each child. Tell them that they will use this bag for their activity today and that they can continue to use this bag for their shopping in the future. Explain that regular

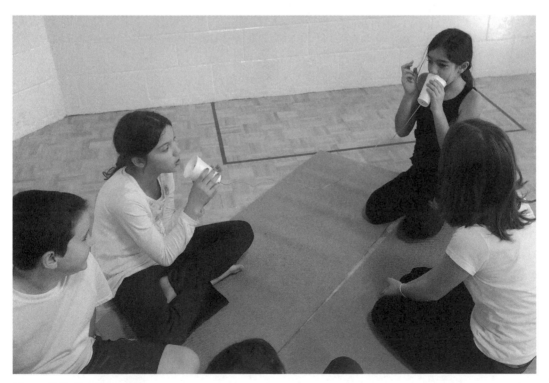

Figure 3.3. Sound waves

plastic disposable bags take up to one thousand years to break down after they are discarded. Set up clues and poses on cards in hoops scattered around the room. These are clues that will help them to save their Earth. Have the children dance to some fast music. When you stop the music, they should visit one of the hoops or "stations" and do the pose that is there and pick up the clue that is there. They should store the clue in their canvas bag. Have them move around the room like this until they have visited every hoop, done the pose that is there, and taken the clue for their bags. At the end you can sit down and read each clue out loud as a group. Some examples of clues are recycle, turn off the water when brushing your teeth, turn down the heat by one degree, donate old clothes and books to thrift stores, take faster showers, plant new plants in the garden, and always turn off the lights when you leave a room. You can add in any additional clues you can think of.

Time: Fifteen to Twenty Minutes

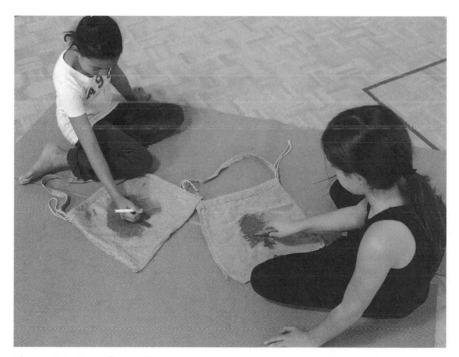

Figure 3.4. Save the earth

Arts and Crafts: The children can draw (using fabric markers) on their canvas bags. They can draw the poses that they visited in each hoop or their visions of how to save the earth.

Time: Fifteen Minutes

Meditation: Ring the chimes now to signal that it is time for the final meditation. Ask the children to lie down on their mats as you dim the lights and put on very soft music. Ask them to lie as still as possible, to close their eyes, and to look at their thoughts. They have thought about many different ways of helping the earth today. With all these ways of preserving the earth, they should be able to picture a beautiful, clean, and healthy Earth in their minds. Tell the children to picture the earth completely free of pollution, with clear blue skies and clean rivers and oceans. Tell them to picture green forests with healthy big trees and sea creatures living in clean water. Tell them to visualize a perfect world. Tell them they can make changes in their lives that will be beneficial to the environment. Allow a few moments of silence and then ring the chimes. Ask the children to begin to wiggle their fingers and toes, arms and legs. They can bring their knees into their chests and wrap their arms around their legs, giving themselves a big hug. They can roll over and come into a seated position.

Time: Five to Ten Minutes

Gratitude: Ask the children to be grateful for themselves and to be grateful that they have the power, knowledge, and energy to save the planet. End with "Namaste, the light inside of me honors the light inside of you."

Time: Five to Ten Minutes

3.

Geometry

Ten- to Twelve-Year-Olds

Educational Elements: Freedom of movement; freedom of choice; self-expression; language enrichment; absorbing abstract ideas in a hands-on, sensorial way; noncompetitive atmosphere

Props: Two large Bristol boards, one for cut outs of shapes for puzzle and one as a control board, Tibetan bowl (or whatever else you would like to use), large easel or blackboard to draw on, marker, yoga mats, music, optional herbal eye pillows

Intention: Strike your Tibetan singing bowl to signal the children to gather in a circle on their mats. Tell them that in class they will talk about geometry. Discuss how geometry is the part of math where they study shapes and angles and measure lengths. Invite discussion from the children. Tell them that they can start by creating some shapes with their bodies.

Time: Five to Ten Minutes

Warm-Up: Tell the children to begin their warm-up by making a ball or circle with their bodies. Then have them stretch right out on the mat on their backs, creating a line. Then have them stand up with legs wide, arms to their sides, creating a triangle. Have them create a few more shapes with their body and then move into a little flow of poses.

Time: Five to Ten Minutes

Connect: Human pyramid. Divide the children into groups of three. Have each group stand in a circle and hold hands. Keeping their feet in the same position, have the children pull their hands together so their heads will begin to come together and their bodies will form a pyramid. Have the children push their hands out so they are now standing straight. Repeat this several times.

Time: Five to Ten Minutes

Activity 1: Guess my shape. Gather the children and invite them to each choose the name of a shape from a hat without showing it to anyone else. They must, in turn, make the shape as best they can by using their bodies. They can pick a partner to help them demonstrate their shape when it is their turn. The other children can guess the names, and as they guess, you can draw them on a large board or easel

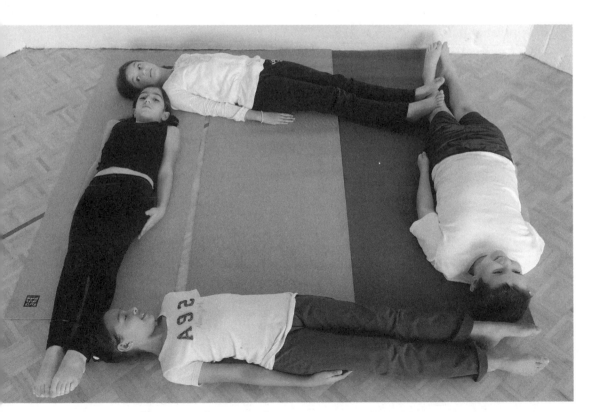

Figure 3.5. Guess my shape

to show them to the class. (Use shapes that are three-dimensional like cylinder, cube, pyramid, rectangular prism, sphere, ellipsoid, ovoid, etc.) The children can later draw all these shapes if they like.

Time: Ten to Fifteen Minutes

Activity 2: Piece the puzzle. Draw a large, multipiece puzzle on Bristol board consisting of triangles, squares, and rectangles of various sizes and then cut them out. Have a "control" Bristol board for later with the original puzzle drawn on it. Each child will receive a piece of the puzzle, and as a group they can work to fit their shapes together. Finally, when they are finished, give them the "control" picture so that they can check to see if they have built the shape correctly. Let them experiment, removing a few pieces of the puzzle to create a new shape. See if they can, for example, use three or four pieces to create a perfect square or a perfect rectangle. Let the children explore.

Time: Ten to Fifteen Minutes

Partner Pose: Have the children work in pairs, and call out names of shapes (e.g., star, moon, or pyramid). Have them work to create these with their bodies.

Time: Five Minutes

Meditation: Strike the Tibetan singing bowl and have the children gather on their mats for their final meditation. Dim the lights, put on soft music, and have the children close their eyes, arms by their sides with palms facing up and chins tilted slightly down to their chests. Ask them to first bring all their attention to their feet. Ask them to tense all the muscles in their feet, hold the muscles tight for four seconds, and then relax all those muscles. Now bring their attention to their calves, and have them tense those muscles for four seconds, then relax them. Guide the children on this full progressive relaxation, which allows them to experience the contrast between tense and relaxed states. Cover each main body area. Then ask them to pull their shoulders up to their ears and then release them. Ask them to scrunch up their faces and then release them and squeeze their eyes and then release them. Now with their whole bodies relaxed, let them lay in silence for a few more minutes, breathing out tension. Ring the Tibetan bowl, and ask them to stretch gradually, roll over to one side, and then come up to a seated position with their eyes closed and hands in their favorite mudra.

Time: Five to Ten Minutes

Gratitude: Ask the children to silently be thankful for all the other children today in class who all worked together to create geometric shapes. They worked together should be proud of their ability to help others and work as a group. They should take this skill and use it in everything they do—at school, at home, and wherever they go. End with "Namaste, the light in me honors the light inside of you."

Time: Five to Ten Minutes

4.

The Food Chain

Ten- to Twelve-Year-Olds

Educational Elements: Freedom of choice, freedom of movement, language enrichment, cooperation, development of a sense of care for the environment

Props: Predrawn cards with either carnivores or herbivores drawn on them, several slips of paper with either "shelter," "food," or "water" written on them, animal pose cards or animal objects, yoga mats, music, chimes, photocopied sheets with predrawn food pyramids for the children to complete and illustrate

Intention: Ring the chimes, bowl, or gong and gather your class together on their mats. Welcome them to yoga. Tell them that they will be discussing nature's food chain in today's class. Ask if they know what this is. Initiate a conversation about the basic needs for animals' survival (food, water, shelter, etc.) and that the animal kingdom is made up of herbivores (plant eaters), carnivores (meat eaters), and omnivores (plant and meat eaters). See if the children can name some and list them on a chart as you go. Illustrate a little food pyramid as your conversation progresses (e.g., grass subsists on sun and water, elk eat grass, lions eat elk).

Time: Five to Ten Minutes

Warm-Up: Tell the children that in the warm-up today, they will do poses of many animals, and as they do them, the children can call out whether the animal is a carnivore, omnivore, or herbivore. Begin a vinyasa of poses.

Time: Five to Ten Minutes

Connect: Feed the animals. Hand out an animal object or animal pose card to each child in the circle. Plan that some of the children will be herbivores (e.g., rabbit, horse, duck, pigeon, butterfly), some will be omnivores (e.g., flamingo, bear, monkey), and some will be carnivores (e.g., wolf, lion, dog). Then place slips of paper in the middle of the circle with the following written on them: a *P* for plant, an *M* for meat, or a *B* for both. Call out the first child's pose in the circle (e.g., rabbit). The child must connect to what his or her animal eats in the corresponding slip (e.g., the rabbit would take a *P* slip). The child should take it back to his or her spot and then do the corresponding pose. Proceed in this way until all the children have had a turn and they have been "fed."

Time: Approx. Ten Minutes

Activity: The survival game. Assign each child in your group a role in this survival game. They can be either an herbivore (mouse, deer, rabbit, etc.) or a carnivore (wolf, cougar, etc.) The children then spread out around the room and assume their roles, moving as their creature would in the wild. Have a supply of papers that read either "shelter," "water," or "food." Place them in a hoop in the center of the room. Turn on fun music and have the children dance. Periodically turn off the music and ask the children to stop each time you do this and take one strip of paper from the hoop. Tell them to choose wisely; they must have enough of each thing to survive, and herbivores need lots of "shelter." When the slips of paper are gone, finish the music and movement part of the game. Now the hunting begins! Ring your chimes and tell the carnivores that they can try to tag an herbivore. Set a time limit on the chasing, and then ring the chimes. If not tagged, the herbivores are safe. If tagged, the herbivore must give their catcher, the carnivore, a "shelter" slip. If the herbivore does not have a "shelter" slip, then they are "eaten" and must sit out. Ring the chimes again and begin a new round. Every few rounds you can yell "drought," "famine," or "attack." Then carnivores only must give up one of their slips (a "water" slip for drought, a "food" slip for famine, or a "shelter" slip for attack). This is how the carnivores can lose all their slips. If they have no more slips left, then they are out. The game ends when the last animal is left standing and is the survivor.

Time: Fifteen to Twenty Minutes

Meditation: Ring the chimes and gather the children for their relaxation, dimming the lights and putting on soft music. The children can stretch out on their mats with their palms facing up, feet out to the sides, and chins tilted slightly down toward their chests. Tell them to slow their breathing and feel their bellies rising on the inhalation and falling on the exhalation. They can imagine now that they are in a forest at dawn. Everything is still and the air is crisp. Tell them to feel the moist dew with their feet as they walk through the forest. Tell them to listen to the crackling leaves beneath their feet. They must be silent so they do not wake the animals. Ask them to notice what they see, to notice that they can see their breath because it is a cool morning. Tell them to imagine touching the soft moss on the logs and the wet leaves on the branches around them. Continue on with this visualization, making it very tactile—have the children use all their senses as they go on their journey. Then enjoy a few silent minutes. Ring the chimes, and ask the children to begin to move and stretch and then roll over and come up into a seated position, hands in their favorite mudras.

Time: Five to Ten Minutes

Gratitude: Ask the children to be silently grateful for the order that exists in our world and to be grateful that the creatures around us all have what they need to survive. We are lucky to have the ability as smart, healthy people to ensure that nature's order does not get interrupted by things like disease, drought, and famine. End with "Namaste, the light in me honors the light in you."

Time: Five to Ten Minutes

5.

De-Stress to Study

Ten- to Twelve-Year-Olds

Educational Elements: Care of self, cooperation, independence, freedom of movement, sensorial exploration, freedom of choice

Props: Material for making herbal eye pillows (fabric, sandwich bags or drawstring bags, beans or rice, dried lavender), yoga mats, music, cutout clock faces made of cardboard (two for each child) with the minutes of an hour drawn on them, scissors for each child, envelopes for children to keep their paper circles in

Intention: Ring chimes or gong, inviting the class to sit on their mats in a comfortable position. Tell them that for class, they will talk about all the things they just can't avoid in life, like tests or exams. But when they get anxious or nervous about these things, they are actually flooding their bodies with chemicals that help them deal with stress. These are their "fight or flight" chemicals. Explain that although these chemicals can give us an advantage in certain situations (when in danger), releasing them all the time will wear them down and make them tired. So they can't let their stress control them or they won't be able to work. Ask the children to talk about stressful situations that they have experienced. Tell them that they will be learning some "de-stressing" tips today that will help them work and study better.

Time: Approx. Ten Minutes

Warm-Up: Ask the children to start by coming up to their knees. Ask them to pretend that it is the end of the day and they have been busy

153

and tense. Ask them to start by giving their loudest lion's roar, sticking out their tongues. This lets out stress. Now bring them into a downward dog pose and have them kick their legs up behind them several times like a horse. This gets their energy out and builds their confidence. Ask them to now stand up. Have them reach into the air as they breath in and then pull down as they exhale, yelling, "Ha!" Have them do this several times. Then begin a vinyasa (see vinyasa 3, page 203).

Time: Five to Ten Minutes

Connect: Group neck massages. Ask the children to come into a circle, and then have each child turn to his or her right and face the back of the child beside them. He or she will give this person a neck and shoulder massage, and the person behind the child will give him or her a massage. Massages are great to do with a loved one when you need a break from studying and you have been seated at a desk for a long

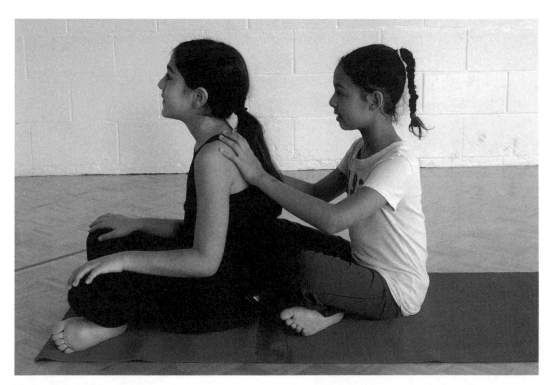

Figure 3.6. Neck massages

time. Ask them to first squeeze their partners' shoulder muscles with two hands, moving back and forth from the neck out to the shoulders. Second, they can put pressure on the back of the person's neck very gently with one hand, moving up to where the spine ends at the skull and then down. Finally, they can place their thumbs on either side of the person's spine just below the neck and then can lean forward and let their body place pressure on the thumbs. Ask them to repeat this a few times. Ask everyone how they feel after their massage.

Time: Five to Ten Minutes

Activity 1: A quiet place. Ask the children to spread out in the room and find a spot where they are not near anyone else. Tell the children that they should have a similar quiet place at home where they can study or think. This is their sanctuary. They need to have this place because school can be loud and crazy. Now that they are in their quiet place in your classroom, they can practice some pranayama, or breathing control work. Ask them to close their eyes and count to five, breathing in with their hands on their bellies. Have them hold the breath for two counts and then exhale for five. Repeat this three or four times. Now encourage them to find a special mantra, or word, that they can repeat to themselves over and over as they exhale: something simple like "Om" or a phrase like "I can do it." Ask them to try this now several times. Let the students know that they can use these techniques at home in their quiet place when they are feeling stressed.

Time: Five to Ten Minutes

Activity 2: Let's prioritize. Hand out a large envelope to each child. Inside they will find a cutout circle with the face of a clock drawn on it. There will also be another identical clock on another circle. This second clock will be cut into pie pieces by the children for this activity. Ask them to imagine that they have sixty minutes to fit in a number of things to do and that they have three items of homework they must complete. Each activity should be cut out from the second clock as a pie piece, the sizes varying depending on how much time they feel they will have to do on each one. They must allow time for a relaxation break and a bathroom break, so have them prepare small pieces to fit into their pie graph. Ask them to think about how big each piece of the pie will be and then cut it out—at the end, all the cut of pie pieces (activities) should fit into the circle and be placed on the first clock, filling the sixty-minute period of time. Afterward, have the students look at each other's pies; they may all be slightly different, depending on how they prioritize their time!

Time: Approx. Fifteen Minutes

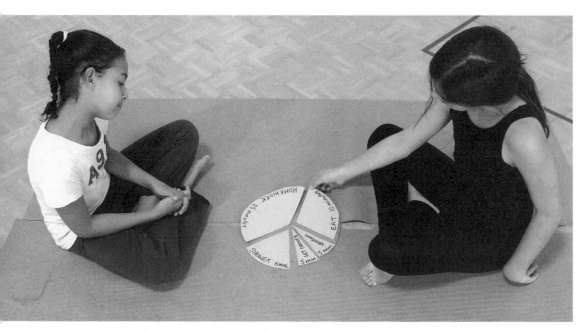

Figure 3.7. Let's prioritize

Arts and Crafts: Herbal eye pillows. These are wonderful for the children to use on their own when they need to rest their eyes and minds and just take a break. Have the children sit in a circle. Give all the children a little cloth bag (you can use drawstring bags from a dollar store, sewn bags that you have made, or even resealable sandwich bags). The top of the bags should remain open and will be either drawn together, sewn, or sealed up in some way at the end of class. Place a large bowl of rice, seeds, or beans mixed with some dried lavender for fragrance in the center of the circle. The children can scoop their own mixtures into their bags, sharing spoons or scoops to do so. When the children are finished, they can help each other seal their bags, or you can come around and seal it for them.

Time: Ten to Fifteen Minutes

Meditation: Ring your chimes or gong, signaling that it is time for the craft to end. The children can use their eye pillows when doing their meditation. Have them lie on their mats. Dim the lights and put on soft music. Ask them to slowly close their eyes to the outside world and begin to look inside their imaginations. Tell them to imagine that they are sitting at the end of a dock on a lake, and the sun is beginning to set. The sun is changing colors: it is yellow at the top, orange through the middle, and red at the bottom where it touches the horizon. Ask them to feel the cool water on their toes as they dangle their feet in the lake. The water is crisp and shiny. Ask them to smell all the smells of the lake and forest: the scent of pine trees and wildflowers. Tell them to feel the air—it is cool and fresh. Ask them to reach down, scoop up a handful of water from the lake, and taste it. Continue with this sensory meditation. After a few minutes of silence at the end, ring the chimes and ask the children to slowly stretch, roll over to one side, and come into a seated position. They can come into bear grip mudra (see page 202). This helps them concentrate when they need to.

Time: Five to Ten Minutes

Gratitude: Ask the children to be silently grateful for opportunities to learn and grow as individuals. They should also be gracious to those that help them along the road in their learning journeys. End with "Namaste, the light in me honors the light in you."

Time: Five to Ten Minutes

6.

The Chakras

Ten- to Twelve-Year-Olds

Educational Elements: Utilizing movement, sensorial exploration of abstract concepts, following a set order, cooperation, reinforcing the importance of "care of oneself"

Props: Copies of a diagram of the body with chakras drawn on it, yoga mats, chimes, music, one chair for each child

Intention: Ring your chimes or Tibetan bowl to signal the start of the class. Invite the children to sit on their mats comfortably. Explain that in today's class they will be exploring the parts of their bodies that the ancient yogis called the chakras. Provide the children a diagram of the body with the chakras. Create this diagram using materials available on the Internet illustrating the chakras. Explain that thousands of years ago, the yogis thought that good health required the free flow of prana or breath energy in between each one of these energy centers or chakras of the body. But explain that it is still true today that if they practice breathing exercises to make their prana flow and do yoga, they can provide their bodies with huge health benefits. When they pay attention to their breath and how this energy flows through them, they are tuning into their chakra system. Show the children each chakra, starting at the root chakra (muladhara), and talk about what organs are located in this area of our bodies.

Time: Ten Minutes

Warm-Up: Explain that they are going to work through a flow of poses that help open up each chakra, getting energy to flow freely through them. Go through the following poses in order (see poses on pages 193–199): the corpse pose, the lotus pose (tell them that this is good for the root chakra), the sailboat twist (this is good for the water chakra), rocking horse (good for fire chakra), camel (for the air chakra), candlestick pose (good for the throat or air chakra), plough pose (also good for air chakra), and the seated forward bend (Venus flytrap pose), which is good for brow or third eye chakra. Finally, lie down in the fish pose, to activate the crown or thought chakra. Have them lie in corpse pose for a moment.

Time: Five to Ten Minutes

Connect: Group balance. Ask the children to form a circle and to take hold of their classmates' wrists on either side of them in the circle. Tell them to all stand up together. Following that, tell them to balance on one foot, and then have them switch to the other foot. They should stay holding on to each other as they all sit back down. Bring to their attention how they helped each other do this. Now ask the children to rub their hands together very quickly to create friction, and after a minute, have them place each palm almost up against the palm of the child on either side of them. Ask them if they can feel this energy between their hands and explain how it connects us all.

Time: Five to Ten Minutes

Activity: Chair poses. Invite the children to sit on chairs placed on their mats. Tell them that you are going to demonstrate how doing chair poses can actually help get energy and breath flowing through their bodies at times when they may be sitting in class with little energy and inspiration. A little chair yoga can get their creative and physical juices flowing and inspire great work! Demonstrate some of the poses on page 161 and have the children think about what chakras the energy in their bodies is flowing through most as they do each particular pose.

Time: Ten to Fifteen Minutes

Partner Pose: Octopus. Invite the children to pair off and do the octopus pose (refer to partner pose 1, page 189). Breathing deeply in this pose will stimulate their fire and water chakras.

Time: Approx. Ten to Fifteen Minutes

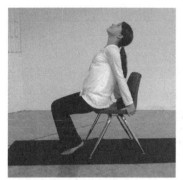

Figure 3.8. Arched back

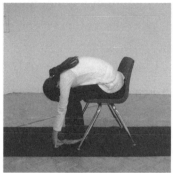

Figure 3.9. Forward bend

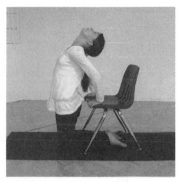

Figure 3.10. Camel

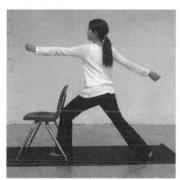

Figure 3.11. Chair warrior

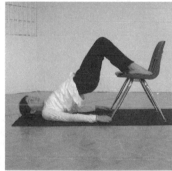

Figure 3.12. Lying shoulder stand

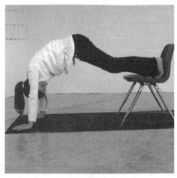

Figure 3.13. Downward dog

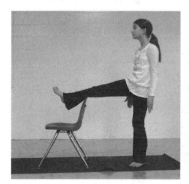

Figure 3.14. Stand and stretch

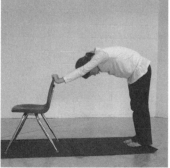

Figure 3.15. Standing fold

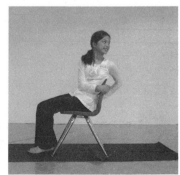

Figure 3.16. Sitting twist

Meditation: Ring your chimes to signal that it is time for the final meditation. Dim the lights and have the children lie down and be still on their mats, with their eyes closed. Put on very soft music. Have them soften their breath. Ask them to breathe in through their noses, and as they do so, feel their breath going all the way down to their root chakra. As the breath reaches their root, tell them to visualize it as a red flame with lots of power and then to breathe out. On their next breath tell them to send that energy down to the water chakra and visualize this area as being orange and fluid, and then tell them to breathe out. Next ask them to inhale down to their fire chakra in their bellies and visualize this area as being very bright yellow, and then tell them to exhale. Next they can inhale deeply down into their air chakra in their heart and visualize it as being a deep emerald green, and then tell them to exhale. Next they can breathe into their throat chakra and feel that it is a very dark blue; then tell them to breathe all the energy out. Then they can breathe into their brow or third eye chakra, right in the center of their heads between their eyes. Ask them to imagine that it is a beautiful purple color and then breathe out. Finally ask them to breathe energy up to the top of the crown of their head and imagine a lighter purple color, almost a light violet, and then breathe out. Ask them to now feel like the breath in their body is flowing evenly wherever it goes, between every chakra. When this energy flows well, they will feel healthy and energetic. Give the children a few minutes of silence and then ring the chimes. Ask them to begin to stretch slowly, roll over onto one side, and then come up into a seated position with their hands on their laps.

Time: Five to Ten Minutes

Gratitude: Ask the children to be thankful that they have the power to activate and understand the energy centers of their bodies and to open them up by using yoga. End with "Namaste, the light inside of me honors the light inside of you."

Time: Five to Ten Minutes

7.

The Earth's Elements

Ten- to Twelve-Year-Olds

Educational Elements: Emphasis on community and mutual respect, freedom of movement and choice, learning about care of the planet, language enrichment

Props: Paper squares, pins and pencils with rubber erasers for the pinwheel craft, book (*Earth, Fire, Water, Air* by Mary Hoffman and Jane Ray), yoga mats, music, several bean bags, chimes, one strap for each child (scarves, belts, or ties can substitute)

Intention: Ring your chimes and gather your group, having them seated on their mats. Welcome them to yoga. Begin a discussion about Earth's elements, asking them if they know what the four main elements are on the planet. They might know that the elements are fire, water, air, and earth. Discuss the powers that each of these elements has, what it can do, and what it provides the earth with. Tell the children that today's activities will show the powers of the elements.

Time: Five to Ten Minutes

Warm-Up: Tell the children that they are going to use straps on their legs today to read an imaginary book. Pass out one strap to each child in the circle (you can use scarves or belts if you like). Have the children lie on their backs on their mats, and have them raise their right legs in the air, knee slightly bent. Tell them to place their straps across the widest part of the foot, holding onto each end of the strap with each hand. As they begin to straighten their legs, have them slide their

163

hands down the straps while still holding tightly. Then they can place both sides of the straps in their right hands and stretch their right legs all the way over to the right side, as if they were opening the cover of a book. They can use their straps to control the stretch. They can then draw the leg back up, pass the sides of the straps into the left hand, and make the leg go all the way over to the left, as if they were turning a page of a book. Have them get used to this motion a few more times, tightening their grip on the strap as they need to increase the stretch. Then have them remove the strap and do the whole process again with the other leg. Afterward, ask them if the insides of their legs feel stretched out.

Time: Five to Ten Minutes

Connect: We can build it. Pass out one bean bag to each child in the circle. Tell them that they must work together to build a huge pyramid. Show them a picture of how the bean bags should look in a pyramid if you would like. One by one ask the children to place a line of bean bags across the floor, then a shorter line on top, then another shorter one on top of that, and so on, until the final child in the circle places the last bean bag right on the very top. Have the children admire the structure that they worked together to build.

Time: Five to Ten Minutes

Activity: Element tag. Explain that in this game everyone will be assigned a role. Two children will be "air." These children will be "it." The rest of the children will be "earth." Explain that when the earth children are tagged by the air children, this will create friction. Friction created by air rubbing earth creates fire, so those who are tagged will be on fire! They must stop when they are tagged and come into a pose (downward dog, triangle, or wide-legged mountain), with enough room for their friends to run underneath them. They remain here (pretending to be on fire) until they are saved. They can only be saved by their friends running underneath their legs like a stream of water. You can tell them that this will put out the fire. Once they are saved they can become earth again and join in the game. Air children can win if they are able to tag all the earth children. Periodically, stop the game and have the children change roles.

Time: Ten to Fifteen Minutes

Breath: Have the children sit down now to cool off after their lively game. Do "blow it out of the water" breathing (see breathing exercise 8, page 206).

Time: Five Minutes

Arts and Crafts: Making a prana pinwheel. Precut an eight-by-eight-inch square of paper for each child and have them fold two opposite corners of their square into the center of the paper. Then slide a pin through the paper's center to hold the corners in place. Place a pencil behind the paper, and have the sharp end of the pin glide right through the paper and into the eraser at the top end of the pencil. This

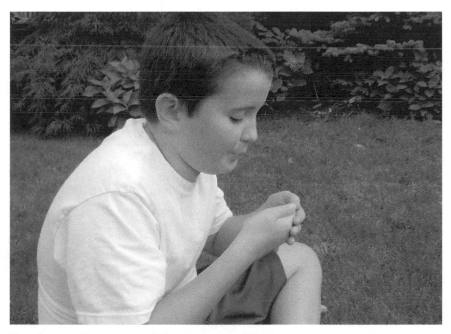

Figure 3.17. Blow it out of the water breathing

will keep the pin in place and attached to the pencil. The children can practice blowing their pinwheels, using strong breaths.

Time: Approx. Ten Minutes

Book: *Earth, Fire, Water, Air* by Mary Hoffman and Jane Ray. This is a fun one for the kids to act out, if time allows.

Time: Five to Ten Minutes

Meditation: Invite the children to lie down on their mats. Dim the lights and put on soft music. Have them close their eyes, with their palms facing up and chin slightly tucked into the chest. Ask them to soften their breath and be aware of every inhalation and exhalation. Tell the children that as they exhale, everything inside of them that they don't want will leave them; it will trickle away, leaving empty space. As they inhale they fill with fresh, happy, light energy. It is like a bright light, filling them up. It will allow them to do anything they want to do. As they breathe out again, all negativity and bad energy leaves; again, as they inhale, positivity and happiness fill them up. Have the children focus on this breathing exercise for a few more minutes and then allow a few minutes of silence.

Time: Five to Ten Minutes

Gratitude: Ask the children to stretch, wiggle their fingers and toes, roll over, and come up into a seated position, with their hands in Venus lock mudra (all the fingers of one hand interlocked into those of the other hand). This connection of the fingers makes them feel warm and loved. Ask the children to be silently grateful for the basics of the earth: fire, air, water, and earth. It is used by us all and connects us.

Time: Five to Ten Minutes

8.

Globe Hopping

Ten- to Twelve-Year-Olds

Educational Elements: Freedom of movement, expression, imagination, sensorial exploration, language enrichment, culture

Props: Photocopied maps of the world (one for each child); pencil, crayons, or markers; pose stamps if you have them, yoga mats, music, chimes, a large globe

Intention: Strike your gong to begin class and have the children relax on their mats. Explain that today they will be traveling around the world and will be discussing all the things there are to see. Invite them to talk about where they have been or would like to go.

Time: Five to Ten Minutes

Warm-Up: Tell the children to begin in a seated position and then reach their arms up to the sky on an inhalation. They should then turn palms outward and press their arms away from themselves, toward the floor on an exhalation. Then have them bring their hands together up in the air, palms pressed flat together above their heads as they inhale. As they exhale, have them lower their arms to either side. Have them do this for a minute and then come to a table top position and begin a vinyasa (see vinyasa 2, page 203).

Time: Five to Ten Minutes

Connect 1: Spin the globe. Have the children seated in a circle and bring out a large globe for them to look at. Have the first child spin the globe and close his or her eyes and then land a finger anywhere on the globe to stop it. For example, that child's finger may have landed on Mexico. That child should do an *M* pose (e.g., mermaid). Pass the globe on to the next child and give him or her a turn. The children will read their spot on the globe where their fingers have landed and do a pose beginning with that letter.

Time: Ten Minutes

Connect 2: Downward dog Chunnel. Ask the children if they know what the Chunnel is. Tell them it is an undersea tunnel that travels from England to France. Discuss the Chunnel with them for a minute, telling them that it is the longest undersea man-made tunnel in the world. It took three years to build, and people travel through it by train. Tell the children that they are going to make their own Chunnel using the downward dog pose. Have the entire group standing in one corner of the room. Invite one child to run to the opposite side of the room and come into a downward dog pose. Then invite the next child to run across, tunnel underneath the first child, and come into his or her own downward dog pose beside the first child. The third child then runs across, tunnels under his or her friends, and creates the third downward dog in the row. Ask the children to run one by one across and create a long "downward dog Chunnel." When the last child has gone through, everyone can rest in the child's pose.

Time: Five to Ten Minutes

Activity: Take a trip. Gather the children in a circle (use chimes to signal this) and tell them that they are taking a trip. They need to help plan how they will get where they are going. Begin at the Atlantic Ocean and move toward Europe. Show them on the globe or map where Europe is. Perhaps they should take a boat to get to Europe. Come into boat pose and row all together. Have the children see different creatures in the ocean and mimic the animal with a pose. For instance, the children can do the dolphin or fish pose. Finally, have them arrive in London. Have the children see Big Ben, followed by an "eyes around the clock" exercise: have them keep their heads still and reach one arm out in front of them with the thumb pointing up. Ask them to make a huge circle with their arm, not moving their heads but following their thumb around the whole circle with their eyes. This is a great eye exercise. Now leave London and perhaps travel by train (you can make a group conga train here) and arrive in Egypt. Everyone can do a pyramid pose. Continue adding to this trip story,

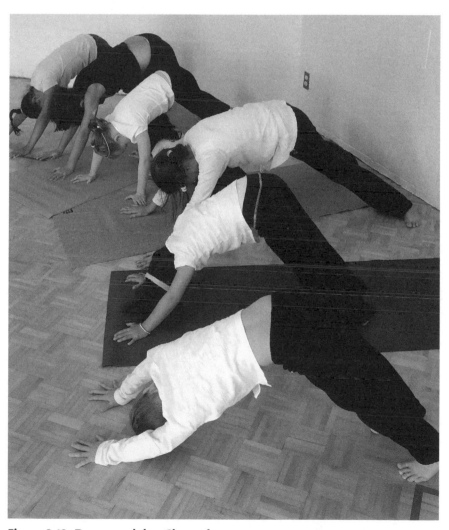

Figure 3.18. Downward dog Chunnel

using poses that the children know, for example, volcano breathing when they reach Hawaii, a seal pose in Antarctica, a camel pose in the Sahara Desert, or mountain pose in the Swiss Alps. The children will have lots of ideas for the story. End up back where you started and have them rest in the child's pose.

Time: Ten to Fifteen Minutes

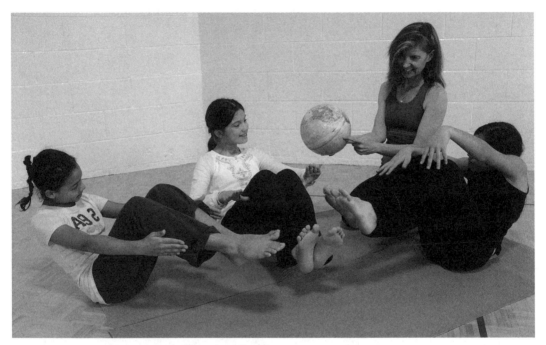

Figure 3.19. Take a trip

Breath: Countdown breath. Have the children relax and sit on their mats. Invite them to do the count the breaths exercise (refer to breathing exercise 15, page 208).

Time: Five Minutes

Arts and Crafts: Where in the world? Give each child a photocopied map of the world. They may draw their journey today using arrows. They can draw or stamp the poses onto their maps that they did at each destination. They can write out the names of the stops as well. Have a master copy labeled with the names for their reference.

Time: Approx. Ten Minutes

Partner Pose: London Bridge. Refer to partner pose 7, page 191.

Time: Five Minutes

Meditation: Ring your chimes to end the art activity and have the children gather on mats for a final relaxation. Dim the lights and put on soft music. The children should lie on their backs with their eyes closed, being as still as they can. Tell them that they are going on a journey on their flying mats. Have them sink down into the mats and feel secure. Have them begin to fly across the world, looking down at the ocean and seeing all the creatures they noticed while on the boat. See the shoreline of Europe and fly over Big Ben and London Bridge. Continue on, feeling the cool air and the fluffy clouds. Continue the journey for a while, ending it when the mats all softly come in for a landing. Give the children a few minutes of total silence, then ring the chimes to end the meditation. Ask them to gradually stretch and roll over onto one side. Ask them to come up to a comfortable seated position and rest.

Time: Five to Ten Minutes

Gratitude: Ask the children to silently think about all the places that they may have seen on their journey today. Ask them to be grateful for all the different kinds of places in the world and the fascinating things to see in each of those places. End with "Namaste, the light in me honors the light inside of you."

Time: Five to Ten Minutes

9.

Fractions

Ten- to Twelve-Year-Olds

Educational Elements: Sensorial exploration and freedom of movement, choice to allow abstract concepts to be absorbed and processed, enrichment of language

Props: Create cards that each illustrate specific parts of whole entities (e.g., one card showing a whole fish and then four separate cards each isolating one specific part of that fish, i.e., gill, fin, etc.), colored modeling clay, yoga mats, chimes or gong, music, herbal eye pillows (optional)

Intention: Gather your class by ringing chimes or striking the gong. Welcome them to yoga, and initiate a conversation about how they are all part of one big united group. For the purposes of this example, let us say you have a class of sixteen children. Tell them that there are sixteen in the class. Everyone is then one-sixteenth of the whole. Ask how many children half the group would be. (Eight.) Ask them how many one-fourth of the group would be. Ask them to stand in groups and then cut that group in half and then in half again. Invite a conversation about fractions.

Time: Five to Ten Minutes

Warm-Up: Begin with the children sitting on their mats. Have them take three big breaths through their nose, and on each exhalation, ask them to say, "Hah," blowing the breath out their mouths. Then begin a vinyasa (see vinyasa 5, page 203).

Time: Five to Ten Minutes

Connect: Orchestra of "hahs." Ask one child to start the orchestra by breathing in and exhaling a "hah." The next child can join in on the next inhalation, so two children now breathe out a "hah." Add in a third child and so on until finally all the children are inhaling and exhaling and repeating "hah" in unison. When this is over ask them to notice what a beautiful, big sound they created together.

Time: Five to Ten Minutes

Activity: Parts of the whole. Present a series of pictures that comprise the parts of an animal (i.e., fish) to the children. The pictures will all be the same but each will have one part of the animal shaded in to highlight itself (e.g., one picture will have the gills shaded, the next picture will have the dorsal fin shaded, the next will have caudal fin shaded, etc.). Explain what the function of each part of the animal is.

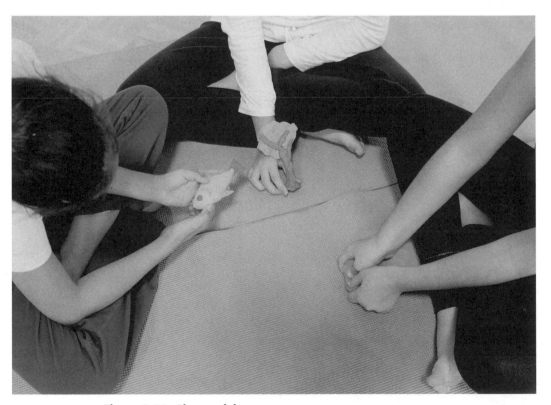

Figure 3.20. Clay models

Discuss which part is for breathing, seeing, swimming, and so on. Ask each child in your group to create one part of the animal (each one of them referring to the picture for guidance) using colored modeling clay. Once finished they can put their pieces together to make one large model of the animal. Discuss how each part of the animal works to help the creature to live, breathe, eat, defend itself, or reproduce. Point out how all the parts work together to create the whole.

Time: Ten to Fifteen Minutes

Meditation: Ring the chimes to signal the end of the class. Invite the children to relax on their mats for a final meditation. Dim the lights and put on soft music. Have them close their eyes, letting their bodies sink into their mats, palms open to the sky. Ask them to feel how the very back of their head feels heavy on the mat. Ask them to let their breath become soft and even. Now ask the children to think of one of the creations that they made today, perhaps a fish, a tree, or a flower. Tell them to visualize this creation. Ask them to picture how colorful it is. Ask them to feel like they can reach out and touch it. How does it feel? Ask them to think about the beauty this thing adds to the earth. After a few minutes of silence, ring the chimes, and ask the children to move and stretch very slowly, to roll over onto one side, and finally to come up into a seated position, with their eyes closed and hands resting gently on their knees. Ask them to notice how they feel.

Time: Five to Ten Minutes

Gratitude: Ring the chimes softly, and tell the children to gradually stretch and roll over onto one side. Ask them to come up to a seated position and bring their hands together in prayer position. Tell them that this hand position is called the prayer mudra (see prayer mudra, page 201). Ask them to close their eyes and take a moment to silently be thankful for everything and everyone around them and for anyone else they love in their lives (things to be grateful for are many, so each class will differ in this way). Then repeat the word "namaste" to them and explain that it means that the "light inside of me bows down to the light inside of you." Have them repeat it. End of class.

Time: Five to Ten Minutes

10.
Healthy Food Choices

Ten- to Twelve-Year-Olds

Educational Elements: Freedom of expression; abstract concepts presented in hands-on, concrete ways; freedom of movement; language enrichment; cooperation; refinement of movement; nutrition

Props: Chimes; mats; photocopies of blank food pyramids; pencils; crayons or markers; small blank cards (eighteen for each child: six green, six yellow, two red, and four blue); colored sticky notes; poster board for each child

Intention: Ring the chimes and signal the beginning of class. Ask the children to gather on their mats for a discussion. Tell them that they have been learning so many poses, breathing techniques, and physical ways to empower themselves in the course so far, but what is equally important is their nutrition. In the history of yoga a great importance has always been placed on a person's diet. It affects not only growth and energy but also mental health and moods. Discuss healthy foods. Invite the children to talk about what meals make them feel energetic. Make a verbal list of essentials to any diet (fruits; vegetables; grains; dairy products; and proteins like fish, soy, and meat). Ask the children how it makes them feel when they eat junk food. Do they feel energized or sluggish? Listen to all the children's input regarding healthy and nonhealthy food, and list the ideas on a chalkboard or paper as you compile ideas and brainstorm.

Time: Five to Ten Minutes

Warm-Up: Have the children in table pose on their mats. Have them alternate between the cow pose, which is where they sink their bellies and look up as they inhale, and cat pose, which is where they arch their backs as they exhale. Then have them begin the vinyasa (see vinyasa 6, page 204).

Time: Five to Ten Minutes

Connect: Squirrels collecting food. Tell the children that they are a group of squirrels that are collecting their food for the winter. Give them each a colored sticky note or a card. Each color should represent a different kind of food (e.g., blue for dairy foods, yellow for grains, green for vegetables and fruits, and red for meats and proteins). There should be a variety of colors divided up and distributed to the children. Now they are ready to burrow. In order to make a tunnel to the burrow, they must create a "downward dog tunnel." Have a board or a container on one side of the room for the child to place their sticky. Have the children stand on one side of the room in a group. The first child then runs to the far side of the room and places his or her sticky on the board. The first child then goes to the downward dog pose, with enough room between their legs for other children to fit, creating the tunnel. The next child then crosses the room, burrows "under" the first, places their sticky on the board, and goes into downward dog in front of the first child, thus adding to the tunnel. The children all take their turns, and when the last child has gone, the children can admire the balanced collection of foods they will have for hibernation that winter!

Time: Five to Ten Minutes

Activity: Create a menu. Distribute eighteen colored cards to each child in the group. Also hand out markers or pencils to all. Tell them that their group of papers represents the number of servings from all the food groups that they need to eat in one day. Each child will get six green and six yellow cards representing the vegetable and grain food groups, two red cards for meat/protein, and two blue cards are for dairy foods. Have each child draw a food from each category on his or her cards. Collect everyone's cards and scatter them around the room in various spots. The children have to create three meals with eighteen cards. Play music and have the children and dance. When it stops, ask them to collect their red protein cards from anywhere in the room and put them on their mats. Have them dance again when the music starts up. When it stops have them collect any four dairy cards and take them to their mats. Continue on in this way until the children have collected all their cards. Ring the chimes and sit with the children. Ask them to divide their cards up into three balanced meals for the day and group them on their mats. Give them a few minutes to do this and then have a discussion about the meals they have created. Give each child a chance to talk about his or her choices.

Time: Approx. Fifteen Minutes

Arts and Crafts: Hand out a blank outline of a basic food pyramid (four food groups: fruits and vegetables, grains, meats and alternatives, dairy and alternatives). The paper outline should be large enough to display the eighteen cards each child has. Ask the children to place their cards in the correct spots on the pyramid to create a nice poster.

Time: Ten to Fifteen Minutes

Meditation: Ring the chimes and have the children lie on their mats in savasana. Dim the lights and put on slow, soothing music. When the children are peaceful, ask them to start thinking about how light and healthy they feel. Talk about the delicious fruits and vegetables that grow on vines, trees, bushes, and fields. Ask the children to visualize these. Ask them to visualize a corn field, a pumpkin patch, or an apple orchard. Give the children beautiful images to visualize as they relax. Then allow them a few minutes of total silence. Ring the chimes. Ask them to bring their knees into their chests, give themselves a big hug, and say something nice to themselves in their minds. Have them roll onto one side and come up to a seated position with their eyes closed and their hands to their hearts.

Time: Five to Ten Minutes

Gratitude: Explain how grateful they must be to have choices in their lives about the food that they eat and for having the power and knowledge to make great choices so that they can grow and feel great. End with "Namaste, the light in me honors the light inside of you." Bow.

Time: Five to Ten Minutes

Appendixes

Book List

Eggbert the Slightly Cracked Egg by Tom Ross

I Know an Old Lady Who Swallowed a Bat by Lucille Colandro

Little Robin's Christmas Vest by Jan Fearnley

Hairy Maclary's Rumpus at the Vet by Lynley Dodd

The Black Book of Colors by Menena Cottin

Ish by Peter Reynolds

My Quiet Place by Douglas Wood

Bringing the Rain to Kapiti Plain by Verna Aardema

My Five Senses by Aliki

The Rainbow Fish by Marcus Pfister

Little Beaver and the Echo by Amy MacDonald

Brown Bear, Brown Bear, What Do You See? by Bill Aartin Jr. and Eric Carle

Dem Bones by Bob Barner

When Sophie Gets Angry—Really, Really Angry by Molly Bang

The Animals' Winter Sleep by Lynda Graham-Barber and Nancy Carol Willis

Children's Atlas of the World by Chez Picthall and Christiane Gunzi

Chickens Aren't the Only Ones by Ruth Heller

A is for . . . ?: A Photographer's Alphabet by Henry Hornstein

Earth, Fire, Water, Air by Mary Hoffman and Jane Ray

Arts and Crafts

1. **Building a Zen garden.** Use small cardboard box lids as bases, with sand and various rocks or shells for filler. A miniature rake can be made with toothpicks, cut and glued together.
2. **Writing with your toes.** Use any size paper you wish and regular-sized markers that will fit easily between the children's toes. Tape the paper to the wall at a reachable distance from the children's feet.
3. **Painting upside down.** Tape paper to the underside of a table or desk and have children lie down underneath on their backs, with their legs in the air. Have paints close by at arm's length. Children can paint with their feet or hands.
4. **Make a lotus.** Use various colors of modeling clay for petals and green modeling clay for the base leaves. Divide large blocks of modeling clay and distribute them equally to the children.
5. **Connections circle.** Make a drawing that looks like a large target with a small circle in the middle surrounded by progressively larger circles. The children should draw themselves in the middle and write or draw those closest to them in the next circle, progressing to the outer circles with members of their school and community, their relatives, their friends, and so on in order of importance to them.
6. **Cardboard puzzles of vertebrates and invertebrates.** Draw these creatures on a large cardboard sheet and cut them out into puzzle pieces that the children will later fit together.
7. **Holiday snowflakes.** Cut silver, red, white, and green pipe cleaners into short and long lengths. Wind the pipe cleaners around each other to create a snow flake. Create some before class as an example for the children.

8. **Pumpkin, witch, or cat Halloween sculptures.** These require blocks of orange, black, and white modeling clay, divided up among the children for them to create scary Halloween sculptures.

9. **Name acrostics.** The children should write their names vertically down one side of a piece of construction paper and then write out the names of whatever poses they can think of horizontally down the page, using the first letters of their names as the first letters of their poses. If they cannot remember the pose names, they can make new ones up.

10. **Body organs.** Using a large roll of paper and fat bright markers, trace your body. The children can use different colors to illustrate the organs, muscles, and so on in the body outline.

11. **Body cutouts.** The children can draw a body, or you can photocopy outlines of bodies for them, and then they can draw what is happening inside (e.g., thinking in the brain area, food in the stomach, air traveling through the lungs, etc.).

12. **Straw painting with your breath.** Use plastic straws. The ends can be dabbed in liquid paints, and children can blow the paint briskly onto papers to make designs. Remind them not to inhale!

13. **Minipuzzles.** Create minipuzzles for each child and draw a pose in each piece. You can usually find cardboard blank puzzles at craft supply stores such as Michael's. Have the children use markers that will not smear.

14. **Modeling clay eight-limbed trees of yoga.** Use brown clay for the tree and use green clay for the leaves. Divide it up before the class so it is ready to hand out quickly.

15. **Yoga man made out of pipe cleaners.** Cut pipe cleaners in half beforehand and distribute three to each child. Have extras on hand.

16. **Mood bead bracelets.** Have the string or wire precut for each child beforehand. They can bead their own bracelets, using colored beads and letter beads, spelling words that describe their mood (e.g., happy, calm, peaceful, energetic, etc.).

17. **Heart necklaces.** Use the hearts that the children have already given out to each other earlier in the class. They can now string them onto a precut necklace string and can even add other beads to them if you wish.

18. **Trust craft.** Paste objects to your cardboard like a sponge, rice, string, or cotton balls. This activity can be done with a partner.

19. **Butterflies.** Drop various shades of food coloring onto dryer sheets to form butterfly images.

20. **Plant a seed.** Plant a seed for the children to cultivate with everything living creatures require. They can also keep a record of when the seed was watered and track its growth.

21. **Make herbal eye pillows.** Use dried seeds or lentils for the stuffing and dried lavender is great for a soothing scent.

22. **Miniskeleton.** Using clay or cardboard, make the bones of the body and connect them to form a miniskeleton. Staple the cardboard or use glue to fasten.

23. **Map of the world.** When globe is spun and a country is chosen, the child does a pose with the first letter of country's name and then draws it where it goes on the map.

24. **"Peace on Earth" Christmas necklaces.** The children can spell the word "peace" with lettered beads and use Christmas-colored beads to decorate the rest of the necklace.

25. **Mandala making.** Use brightly colored markers for this work.

26. **Vinyasa-stamped strips.** It helps to have a variety of colored stamp pads, with a few stampers placed at each, so the children can share and not all be using the same stamp pad.

27. **Yin-yang person.** Draw both sides of yourself with a line down the middle using person-shaped paper.

28. **Passport.** Children stamp the passport at each stop during a freeze dance session.

29. **Prana pinwheel.** Use square-shaped paper and very sturdy straws or pencils.

30. **Polygons.** Using straws that connect gradually, the children

name the different polygons (e.g., pentagon) and then add to them, forming different shapes.

31. **Parts of the animal.** When using the toy animals to learn poses, have them make a mammal, fish, reptile, bird, or amphibian and name the parts of each.

32. **Land and water forms (island, lake, peninsula, cape, bay, archipelago, gulf, etc.).** Children act these out these forms with others acting as the water that flows around the landforms.

33. **Emotion faces.** Children can draw different expressions on a large sheet of paper with blank faces on it.

34. **Yoga word search.** You can make this beforehand and photocopy it for the children. Include language you have used in your previous classes.

35. **"Balance" figure.** Make a "balance" figure when doing a class about balancing your life—for example, a stick man on a stand that pivots.

36. **Utopia puzzle.** The children add ideas of what the perfect world would look like (using a giant Bristol board).

Partner Pose Guide

1. Octopus. One child lies down on his or her back and spreads out his or her legs and arms to form four legs of the octopus. The next child lies over the first, on his or her back as well, spreading arms and legs out to form four more of the octopus's legs. They have now created the eight legs of the octopus.

2. Shoulder wheels. The children stand up side by side and join hands. They slowly begin to draw a big circle in the air, keeping their arms close together. This gives the muscles around the shoulder sockets a good stretch. After they have done some forward circles, they can try going backward. They can then switch around and do it with their other two arms connected.

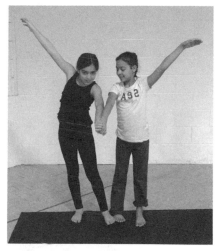

Partner Pose 2. Shoulder wheels

3. Row your boat. The children sit facing one another and connect their hands. They bring the soles of their feet together and gradually lift their feet up off the ground, balancing on their sitz bones. When they feel balanced, they can begin to row the boat, taking turns leaning forward and backward.

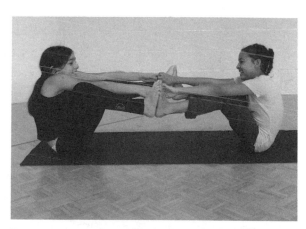

Partner Pose 3. Row your boat

4. Double downward dog. One child goes into a downward dog pose. The second child comes into a table top pose in front of the first (on hands and knees) and then carefully puts his or her feet, one at a time, on the shoulders of the first child, and pulls into a raised-looking downward dog pose. The children then switch positions.

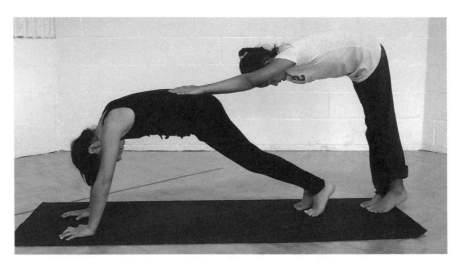

Partner Pose 4. Double downward dog

5. Table and chair. One child goes down on hands and knees, forming a table position. The second child then goes into chair pose and slowly tucks his or her knees under the "table."

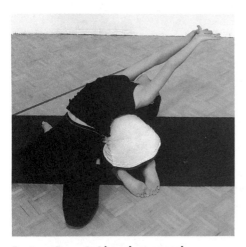

6. Lizard on a rock. One child crouches into a tight little rock on the floor. The second child sits down beside the rock and leans over it, coming into a backward bend, looking up to the sky, arms out, over the first child as if he or she is a lizard basking in the sun on a rock.

Partner Pose 6. Lizard on a rock

7. London Bridge. The children stand a few feet apart, facing each other. The first child lifts his or her right leg, and the second child holds the first child's ankle with his or her left hand. The first child then puts his or her right hand on the second child's shoulder to help balance. The second child then lifts his or her right leg, and the first child holds the lifted ankle with his or her left hand. The second child holds onto the first child's shoulder for balance. As they are doing this tell them that they are the London Bridge, raising the bridge for the ships to pass underneath.

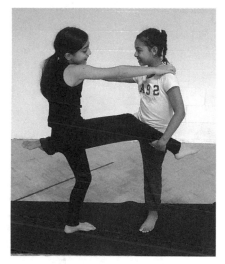

Partner Pose 7. London Bridge

8. Twist and turn. The children sit cross-legged in front of their partner with their knees touching. They each put their right hands behind their backs, and with their other hands, they grab their partner's left hand. They take a big breath, and as they breathe out, they twist away from their partner, looking over the partner's right shoulder. They can do this several times.

9. Partner tree. The children stand side by side. Tell them to gradually feel one foot sinking heavily into the earth like roots reaching into the ground. The other foot feels lighter and gradually lifts off of the ground. The children can then rest the sole of that foot on their calf or even on their inner thigh (not their knee). The children can then hold onto each other with one arm for balance. Have them sway like trees blowing in the wind.

10. Hot lava. The children begin by sitting back to back and link their arms. Tell them they are lava at the bottom of the volcano. They then should lean on each other to rise up like the boiling lava rising to the top of the volcano. Gradually, the children work together to stand up.

11. The box. One child lies on his or her back with the child's legs raised and the soles of his or her feet flat. The second child lays his or her tummy on the first child's feet and reaches for that child's hands. When the child feels balanced, the first one lifts the second off the floor, having that child come into a kind of flying airplane pose. Then ask them to make themselves into a square shape. The flying child can lean his or her head down and lower his or her legs so that the two children together form the shape of a box. They can then switch places.

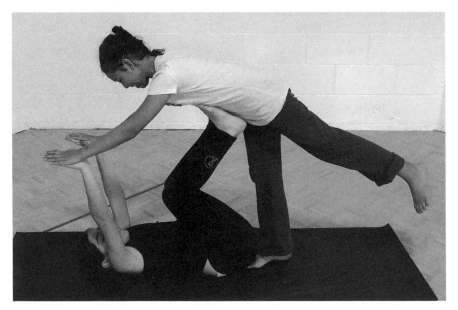

Partner Pose 11. The box

12. Taffy pull. Have the children face each other and hold onto each other's right wrist with their right hand. Have them then step back two or three feet and bend their knees, squatting down a bit, thighs parallel to the floor. They then pull their right hip back, stretching out the right side of their bodies. They will pull each other naturally back and forth. Tell them they are making taffy. Have them then switch arms and stretch on the other side. This is a great side body stretch.

Poses
Sea Creatures

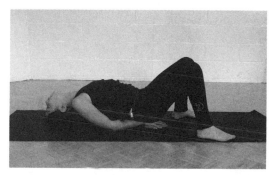

Fish

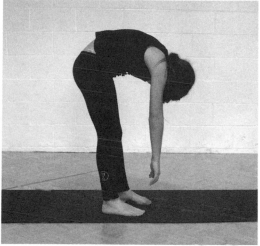

Octopus

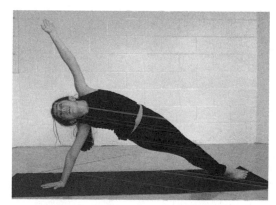

Mermaid

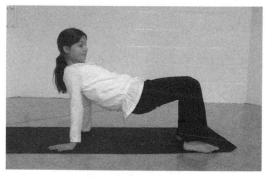

Crab

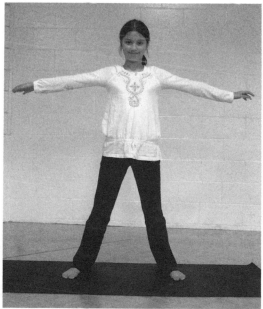

Starfish

Birds

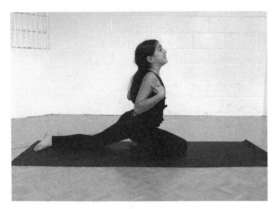

Pigeon

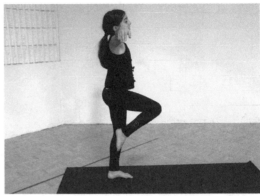

Stork

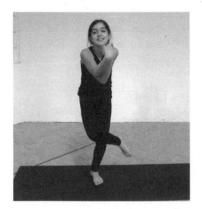

Eagle

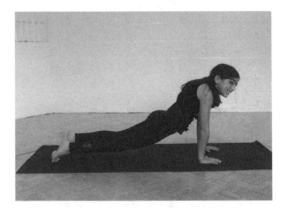

Peacock

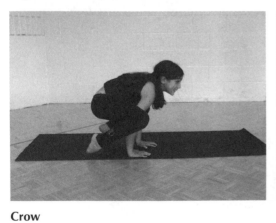

Crow

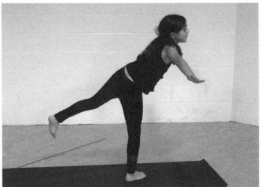

Flamingo

Mammals

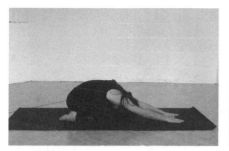

Child's pose

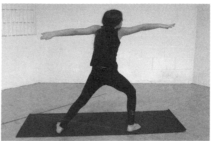

Warrior

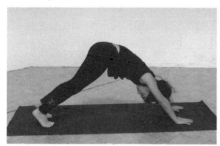

Dog

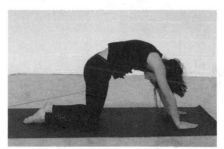

Cat

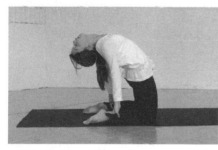

Camel

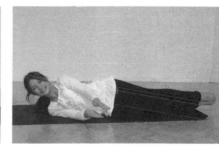

Seal

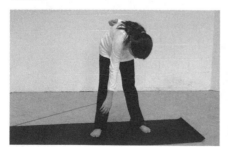

Elephant

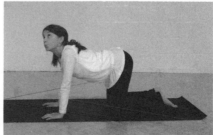

Cow

Amphibians and Reptiles

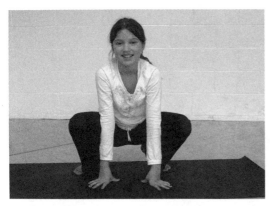

Frog or toad

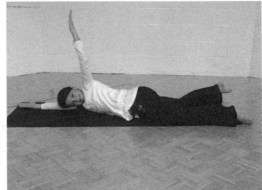

Alligator

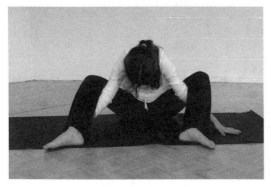

Turtle

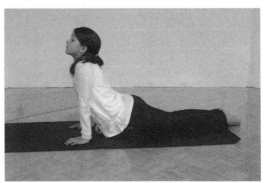

Snake

Insects

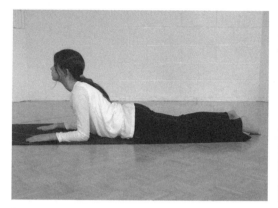

Locust

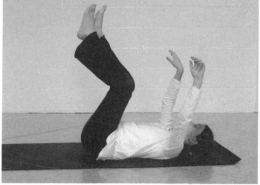

Dead Bug

Vegetables

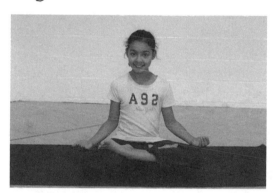

Lotus

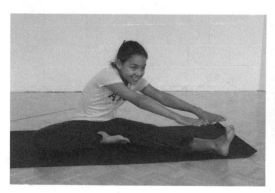

Venus flytrap

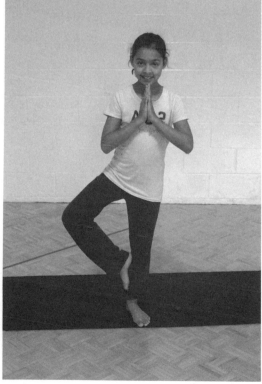

Tree

Minerals

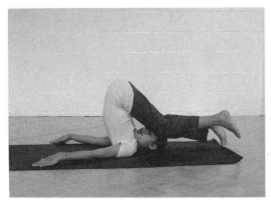

Plough

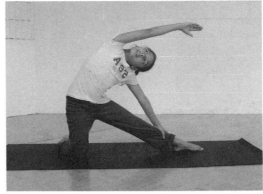

Gateway

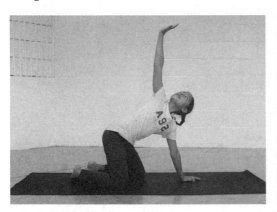

Needle and thread

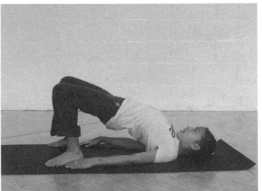

Bridge

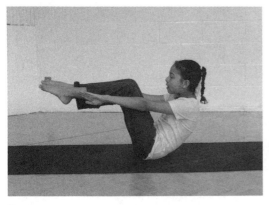

Boat

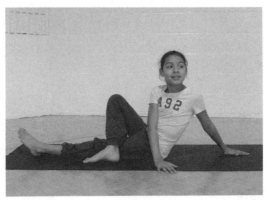

Sailboat

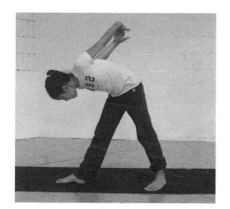

Pyramid

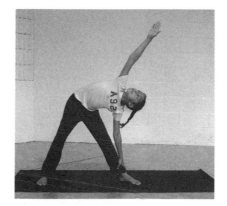

Triangle

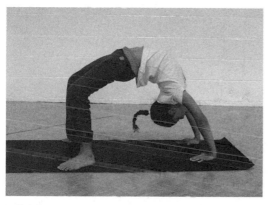

Wheel

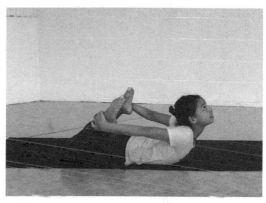

Rocking horse

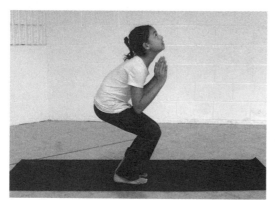

Chair

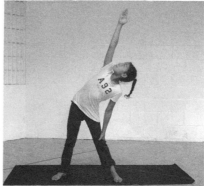

Moon

Mudra Guide

Mudras are hand and finger gestures used in yoga. When performed they are said to seal and direct certain energies within our bodies. The purpose of mudras in this program is not only to introduce them to kids as an interesting and fun concept but also to allow children to, by practicing them, reach a more relaxed, quiet state. They can therefore feel settled and more receptive to the content of the class going on around them. Mudras are simply just fun for kids; they are like doing yoga with their hands! The following are a few that are used in this program:

Prayer mudra. This is done by bringing the palms of the hands together in a prayer position. Tell the children that this mudra shows that we respect each other. It also makes us feel balanced.

OK mudra. This mudra is done by pressing the thumb up against the index finger. Tell the children that this makes us feel "OK"—it sharpens our minds and helps us think.

Earth mudra. This is done by pressing the ring finger up against the thumb. Tell the children that this mudra helps make them feel patient and responsible.

Water mudra. This is done by pressing the baby finger up against the thumb and extending the other three fingers straight up. The hand now looks like a waterfall, falling into a pond. Tell the children that this mudra helps keep all the water that is inside our bodies balanced and flowing.

Tall house mudra. This is done by pressing the middle finger up against the thumb, which forms a shape that looks like a house with a pointy roof. Tell the children that this mudra helps all the joints and muscles in our bodies work well.

Pond mudra. This is done by having both hands resting in front of us. The palms are facing up, with one hand resting in a cradled position in the other one. This looks like a pond. Tell the children that when they look down into this pond, they can take all their negative thoughts and let them trickle down into it, one by one. Then when the thoughts are nestled on the pond, they can simply blow them away.

Bear grip mudra. This is done by extending the left palm out from the body, with the thumb down. Make a little hook out of your hands by pressing your fingers tightly together and curving them down. Bring the right hand over top of the left, hooking the fingers into those of the left hand. When you try to pull your fingers apart you, will see that they have a "bear grip" on each other! Tell the children that this mudra helps them concentrate hard when they really need to.

Venus lock mudra. This is done by interlacing all the fingers of one hand into those of the other hand. Tell the children that Venus was the goddess of love, and when we connect our fingers together it is as if they are all loving each other. It makes us feel warm and loved.

Suggested "Vinyasas" (Warm-Up Flows)

Vinyasa 1. Mountain / crescent moon (left side) / mountain / crescent moon (right side) / standing starfish / flamingo / downward dog / flamingo (other leg) / downward dog / newt / kayak / alligator / table / cat / cow / cat / cow / crow / lotus.

Vinyasa 2. Butterfly / Venus flytrap / wheel / corpse / sit / table / downward dog / mermaid (one side) / downward dog / mermaid (other side) / newt / downward dog / warrior (left leg forward) / mosquito / downward dog / warrior (right leg forward) / mosquito / downward dog / sit / roll in a ball / dead bug.

Vinyasa 3. Mountain / jellyfish / elephant / mountain / triangle (right leg) / mountain / triangle (left leg) / mountain / goddess / downward dog / lunge forward (left leg) / downward dog / lunge forward (right leg) / downward dog / newt / table / cat / cow / cat / cow / child's pose.

Vinyasa 4. Corpse / bridge / corpse / sit cross-legged / butterfly / camel / gateway (left leg out) / camel / gateway (right leg out) / downward dog / mountain / jellyfish / warrior (right leg first) / mountain / warrior (left leg first) / tall mountain / tree (one leg) / mountain / tree (other leg) / downward dog / newt.

Vinyasa 5. Child's pose / table / cat / cow / cat / cow / downward dog / raise leg / pigeon (one side) / downward dog / raise other leg / pigeon (opposite side) / downward dog / mountain / warrior (left side) / mountain / warrior (other side) / downward dog / frog / sit / lotus / turtle / candlestick / plough / roll like a ball / corpse pose.

Vinyasa 6. Sit / forward neck rolls (side to side) / rub temples with index fingers / rub cheeks / wiggle ears / eagle arms / bend forward / come up / reverse eagle arms / bend forward / arms up to sky / relax them down / boat / sailboat (one leg) / sailboat (other leg) / turtle / downward dog / mountain / eagle / mountain / eagle (other leg) / mountain / downward dog / legs go back, lower body down / snake / rocking horse / child's pose.

Breathing Exercises

1. **Bunny breathing.** Deeply exhale through the mouth, then with the mouth closed, take three short, quick inhalations through the nose, crinkling the nose up like a bunny's. Exhale deeply through the mouth, and take three more quick inhalations through the nose. Repeat.

2. **Hoberman sphere breathing.** With the mouth closed, hold the Hoberman sphere up in front of you at chest height. As you breath in, open up the sphere, while at the same time expanding your own belly and chest, mimicking the motion of the sphere. As you exhale, close the sphere with your hands, emphasizing the emptying out of air from the body. Repeat.

3. **Alternate nostril breathing.** With your right hand in front of your nose, take a big inhalation, and as you exhale, cover the right nostril with the right thumb. Pause, then breath in through the left nostril. Pause, then cover the left nostril with the ring finger of the right hand, and exhale fully. Repeat this process a few times.

4. **Take your animal for a ride breathing.** Lying on your back in corpse pose, have the stuffed toy evenly balanced on your stomach. As you inhale deeply through the nose, observe how your belly rises and fills up, allowing the toy to rise. Then observe how the toy lowers down smoothly upon exhalation. Even breathing is required with this exercise as well as mindfulness so that the toy does not fall off.

5. **Straw breathing.** Exhale fully through the mouth, then stick your tongue out and curl it into a straw shape. Inhale fully through the mouth, as if you are sipping air through a straw. Close the mouth and exhale through the nose. Repeat.

6. **Bee breathing.** This breath draws awareness to the vibrational sound made with each exhalation. Inhale deeply through the nose, then with the mouth slightly open, exhale while at the same time making a buzzing sound with your tongue, like the sound of a bee. Inhale through the nose and repeat.

7. **Volcano breathing.** Lower your body down into a squatting position, with hands together to your heart. Deeply inhale through the nose, and imagine that lava inside you is rising up to the top of your head, ready to erupt. As you inhale rise up to a standing position, and as you exhale through your mouth, raise your arms up to the sky as if the volcano is erupting. Lower and repeat this several times. This is a great breath for letting off steam and energy.

8. **Blow it out of the water breathing.** Sitting cross-legged, bring your palms together in front of your belly. Your palms should be facing up, one on top of the other to form a cup shape. This will be your imaginary pond. Begin to think of any negative thoughts you may have or any worries or anxieties. Collect these in your mind, inhale through your nose, and exhale vigorously through your mouth into your little pond. Imagine that all the negative thoughts in your mind have been blown away across the pond. Repeat.

9. **The giving breath.** Sitting cross-legged and have your palms on top of your knees, facing up. Inhale through your nose, and at the same time raise your right palm up to the sky. On the exhalation, place that palm on your chest, over your heart. As you inhale, imagine that you are filling your palm up with all the goodness in your heart and open your arm out away from your chest, as if you are sending goodness out to the world. As you exhale, slowly lower that arm down, placing the palm back on top of your knee. Repeat this on the other side with your left hand.

10. **Grab the sky breath.** Come to a standing position with legs spread shoulder width apart. As you inhale deeply through the nose, reach up with your right hand to the sky, as if you are grabbing it. As you exhale through your mouth, bring that hand to your heart. Repeat this on the other side. This is a vigorous, energizing breath.

11. **Om breath.** In a seated position, close your eyes and draw your attention fully to the sound of your breath. Inhale through the nose, and begin a long drawn out exhalation through the mouth while saying, "Om." Pause and listen to the silence. Then inhale through the nose and repeat at least three times. This breath is excellent for clearing the mind and bringing one's focus inward.

12. **Synchronized breathing with neck rolls.** In a seated position, relax your arms and shoulders fully. Close your eyes. Inhale through your nose, and as you exhale, drop your head down toward your right shoulder. As you inhale, let your head move to the left slowly, toward your left shoulder. Pause. As you exhale, have your head sweep back toward the right shoulder. Repeat. Notice how each breath is synchronized with a movement.

13. **Growing breath.** Come to child's pose on the floor. Inhale and exhale fully through the nose. As you inhale through the nose, raise your head slightly, and then exhale. On your next inhalation raise your shoulders up, and then exhale. On your next inhalation come to standing on your knees, and then exhale. On your next inhalation bring one foot flat to the floor, and then exhale. On your next inhalation bring both feet flat to the floor so you are standing. Continue in this way, synchronizing each breath to a movement, until you are fully grown, like a giant tree with arms stretched up to the sky.

14. **Darth Vader breathing.** In a seated position, close your mouth and exhale fully through the nose. Place your tongue to the roof

of your mouth, and try to constrict your throat a little. This will allow you to hear your breath. Breathe deeply through your nose, and as you exhale through the nose, listen to the breath in your throat. You can liken it to the sound of Darth Vadar's breath. You can also hear that it sounds like the waves on the ocean. This breath is done with the mouth firmly closed.

15. **Count the breaths.** Come to a seated position. Exhale fully through the mouth. Raise your hand out in front of you and make a fist. Inhale through the nose. As you exhale through the nose open up one finger from your fist. Repeat this breath five times until your fist is fully open. You can repeat with the other arm if needed. This exercise is good for bringing the group back to focus after a vigorous activity.

About the Author

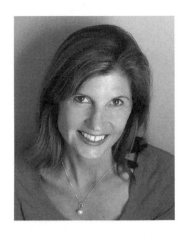

A graduate of Queen's University in Kingston, Ontario, ADRIENNE RAWLINSON is a certified Montessori teacher and registered yoga teacher. She studied yoga under Maureen Rae in Toronto and Erich Schiffmann in Chicago. Knowing that she wanted to offer the gift of yoga to children, she put together her program, drawing from her yoga and Montessori teaching experience, and she began offering afterschool and weekend workshops to children in her area. She currently teaches Montessori and yoga in Oakville, Ontario.